Sleeping Like a Baby

Pinky McKay is the bestselling author of *100 Ways to Calm the Crying*, *Toddler Tactics*, *Parenting by Heart* and *Sleeping Like a Baby*, all of which are endorsed by the Australian Breastfeeding Association and La Leche League International. *Sleeping Like a Baby* and *100 Ways to Calm the Crying* are also endorsed by the Australian Association of Infant Mental Health.

An International Board Certified Lactation Consultant and a sought after guest and keynote speaker, Pinky has spoken across Australia, New Zealand and the United States, as well as presenting a TEDx talk 'Surrender is not a Dirty Word'. She's an expert source, she writes for national and international publications including Essential Baby, HuffPost Parents and *Daily Mail* and is a frequent guest on TV, appearing on *Today*, *Weekend Sunrise*, *A Current Affair* and *The Project*.

Pinky's gentle parenting techniques offer effective alternatives to 'baby training approaches', which may have long-term negative effects on infants' emotional and mental health, result in premature weaning from breastfeeding, and undermine parents' confidence and connection with their little ones. Her real-world experience stems from being a mother of five and a grandmother of three.

pink

D1362026

ALSO BY PINKY McKAY

Toddler Tactics

100 Ways to Calm the Crying

Parenting by Heart

Sleeping Like a Baby

PINKY McKAY

Australia's calm baby expert

PENGUIN BOOKS

PENGUIN BOOKS

UK | USA | Canada | Ireland | Australia
India | New Zealand | South Africa | China

Penguin Books is part of the Penguin Random House group of companies
whose addresses can be found at global.penguinrandomhouse.com.

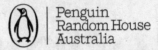

Penguin
Random House
Australia

First published by Penguin Group (Australia), 2006
This edition published by Penguin Random House Australia Pty Ltd, 2016

Design by Laura Thomas © Penguin Random House Australia Pty Ltd
Cover photograph by Olesia Bilkei/Shutterstock.com
Typeset in Adobe Caslon by Laura Thomas
Colour separation by Splitting Image Colour Studio, Clayton, Victoria
Printed and bound in Australia by Griffin Press, an accredited ISO AS/NZS 14001
Environmental Management Systems printer.

National Library of Australia
Cataloguing-in-Publication data:

McKay, Pinky, 1952– author.
Sleeping like a baby / Pinky McKay.
9780143573340 (paperback)
Crying in infants.
Comforting of infants.
Parent and infant.

649.122

penguin.com.au

For all the parents who are soothing wakeful babies and feeling alone in the darkness of night-time, sleep deprivation and self-doubt. Hold and cuddle and listen to your baby. Trust yourself – you have got this!

I do not love him because he is good, but because he is my little child.

Rabindranath Tagore

A note from the author
Because children come in both genders, I have
alternated the terms 'he' and 'she' throughout
this book – no sexism intended. Boys and girls
have equal ability to cause sleepless nights and,
whether baby boy or girl, are equally delightful,
day and night!

Contents

Introduction

There is perhaps nothing more delicious than gazing at a sleeping baby, watching her tiny rosebud lips curl into an involuntary grin, or listening to her gentle sighs. Sadly though, in our culture the standards bar for infant sleep has become so high that, for many parents, the words 'sleeping like a baby' are fraught with anxiety that is spilling into every aspect of their lives.

Each day, I receive more emails and Facebook messages than I can respond to from parents asking for advice on gently helping their babies and toddlers to sleep. Many parents feel pressured that they are creating dependency or lifelong problems by not 'teaching' their baby to sleep. There also seems to be increasing pressure to make even happy babies sleep more often and for longer.

Instead of having the confidence to accept that even though my son, who is now eighteen weeks old, isn't

*a 'textbook' baby, I was ignoring how happy he is and
how well he is thriving. I kept wanting him to nap longer
by day even though he was sleeping pretty well at night.
I was so confused I didn't know which way was up. I
was feeling guilty that I was 'accidental parenting' and
ultimately harming him – robbing him of learning the
skills he needed.*

Sandra

It can seem as though every single person you meet – even
perfect strangers – want to know, 'Is he sleeping through?'

*He's delicious. He smells like rainbows. He's the best
thing I've ever done (along with my bigger baby). He
smiles this gummy smile when he looks up at me. His
hair is so soft. His cheeks are so fat. He is so perfect I
want to have ten of him. Who gives a rat's arse about
whether he sleeps X hours at a time yet? He just got
here. Just stare at him for a while. Welcome him! He's
perfect, isn't he?*

Emily

If you have a wakeful baby, it can seem as though you have
only two options. She can undergo sleep training, which
means leaving your baby to cry, often for hours; or you
have to just 'suck it up' and stagger around in a zombie-like
state without support because 'this is your choice'.

I am the first to agree with you that it is helpful to
have practical strategies to settle your baby so he (and
you!) can sleep better within the realm of what is

normal and healthy – and you can do this without tears. However, too often the only options offered to parents are versions of 'cry it out' or 'controlled crying'. Many of these programs include rigid feeding and sleep routines that deny the needs of babies for touch and comfort as well as food, as parents struggle to make their baby fit the advised timetable. These strict regimes can set parents up for failure. As they strive to achieve the mythical 'good baby' who self-settles (or stops signalling) and sleeps all night without stirring, many parents silently wonder, are we doing something wrong? Or do we have a particularly difficult baby?

> When I was pregnant a friend recommended a book that is all about routine, routine, routine. Wanting to do the best for my baby, I tried implementing a routine in the first few weeks, without success. I felt like a failure.
>
> I would get frustrated when my little princess woke 'early' from a nap or didn't want a feed at the prescribed time, or worse, wanted to feed earlier than the routine would tell me to expect. After a few blessed weeks of her sleeping from 7 p.m. to 5 a.m. with a dream feed, she started waking again for a night-time feed. I thought, gee, I must really be getting things wrong!
>
> I met a fellow mum for coffee yesterday and she mentioned how wonderful your book Sleeping Like a Baby is. On a whim, I picked up a copy and could not put it down! Even after the first few chapters, I realised that the only thing I've been getting wrong is my attitude. Instead of getting frustrated that my beautiful baby isn't

doing what I want her to do, I realised that I'm not doing what she needs me to do. What a light-bulb moment! Not only that, but I realised that in terms of her settling and sleeping in general, we're doing a great job.

Last night when she woke for a feed in the wee hours, I snuggled in with her. I felt grateful that I could breastfeed my precious little bundle and enjoyed that peaceful moment – I didn't flick through Facebook, emails or Pinterest like I usually would. I just enjoyed being close with my baby. Yesterday and today I made a conscious effort to really observe her, respond to her cues and connect with her. She usually has a very grumpy and unsettled period late in the afternoon, but instead she was happy, playful and a joy to be around.

I'm sad that I've wasted the last four and a half months trying to fit my baby into a mould instead of embracing who she is.

Kara

Your baby is not a cardboard cut-out who can be expected to fit a feeding and sleeping template according to his approximate age. When you struggle to impose imprecise strategies onto your unique baby, you risk severing the connection between yourself and your child (or never really making it). You may even start to feel resentment and ambivalence towards your baby as your instincts to comfort him are torn against advice not to 'give in'.

Simplistic, 'one size fits all' sleep training approaches don't take into account that as well as the more obvious needs to be kept clean and fed, babies and children have legitimate emotional needs for comfort and security. Optimum infant brain development depends on responsive interactions between infants and their carers and sensory input, including touch, movement and eye contact. In our eagerness to achieve the solitary-sleeping, self-soothing infant, we have lost sight of the most basic baby need: to develop trust and form loving relationships. This process – attachment – is a behavioural system that operates twenty-four hours a day, even when your baby is asleep, which could be (with luck) up to 60 per cent of the time. It isn't justifiable to respond to a baby during daylight hours and then neglect his needs when the sun goes down.

Each baby is a unique and very special little person and you are the expert on your individual child. Therefore, I would like to introduce you to a stress-free approach to infant sleep that will encourage confidence in your parenting skills *and* a strong connection with your baby.

I believe that one of the best skills any parent can learn is how to read your baby's non-verbal cues so you know not only when is the best time to encourage sleep, but also when your baby will be most receptive to playing and learning, when she is hungry and when she just wants some quiet time. This way, you can organise your day to fit your baby's needs as well as your own, without the frustration of power struggles over sleep. You can also give your baby cues so that learning to sleep becomes a two-way process of communication between you both. By learning your baby's language as well as simple ways to encourage sleep that will not result in tears (for you or your baby), you will be able to solve your baby's sleep puzzle. This is both efficient and effective: you will be more skilled and your baby will be more adaptable – she will not depend on being in her own bed in a darkened room at certain predetermined times every single day, and your life won't revolve entirely around your baby's sleep.

Sleeping Like a Baby will help you understand infant sleep at each stage of development and how your baby's development can affect his behaviour, including sleep. I will also show you how to create a safe sleeping environment, how to read your baby's cues so that you can enhance bonding and development as you help him learn to sleep, how infant feeding patterns and nutritional needs can influence sleep, how you can elicit a relaxation response by using non-invasive aids such as music, massage (for infants and toddlers) and meditation (for toddlers), how to encourage sleep that is appropriate to your child's stage of development and how to make changes gradually with love, when you and your baby feel ready.

One of the biggest issues around infant sleep is creating 'bad habits'. Parents ask, 'If we take our baby into our bed, or give him a dummy, or allow him to settle in a sling or on the breast, how will we ever get him to settle and sleep alone?' *Sleeping Like a Baby* addresses these issues and shows you how to gradually change any habit at any stage, with love, not tears, and how to gently introduce new sleep arrangements as your baby grows.

Sleeping Like a Baby includes stories from parents because I believe that when we feel safe to share how our babies and toddlers really behave and how we honestly feel, we can learn from each other. Hearing about others' experiences can validate our own feelings and 'failings', as it demonstrates the uniqueness of each baby and family without alienating anybody.

I dislike labels because they can set parents up for failure or feelings of exclusion when their parenting styles don't fit neatly within precise definitions. I would argue that attachment, for example, is not a parenting style, but a basic need of every child, regardless of how it is fed or where it sleeps, and all parents need support whatever their lifestyle choices. *Sleeping Like a Baby* therefore embraces a range of gentle, responsive baby-care techniques that don't necessarily fit labels. However, I do offer support and information to parents who choose options such as a baby-led approach to sleeping and 'extended breastfeeding' (another label I dislike since it implies a deviation from what is natural and normal, depending on your interpretation).

As an International Board Certified Lactation Consultant, I also unapologetically acknowledge breastfeeding as optimum infant nutrition and the biological norm. In my experience, much confusion arises for parents when infant sleep expectations are based on what may indeed be deemed normal for a formula-fed baby, but have little relevance to a breastfed baby who will want to breastfeed for comfort, an immune boost if he has been exposed to bugs (transfer of saliva from baby to mother's breasts signals your body to produce antibodies to bugs your baby has been exposed to), or because he needs to signal his mother's breasts to make more milk during a growth spurt or developmental leap. This confusion can lead to early weaning, as confidence about your milk supply is unnecessarily undermined.

Sleeping Like a Baby will help you relax and enjoy your baby without being obsessed about sleep – hers or yours! It will help you to understand the association between infant sleep and optimum development, in particular infant brain development and emotional development, and how, by creating a healthy sleep environment that affirms the whole child, you will be creating a healthy attitude to sleep that will last beyond infancy.

You will gain much more than just a good night's sleep in the process: your confidence will develop as you learn valuable skills and your connection with your child will be strengthened. You will be making a long-term investment in your child's development as well as his attitude to sleep and you will feel empowered.

The con of controlled crying

‘I spent so much time trying to teach my first baby to sleep. I wished I'd spent it enjoying him.’

Megan

Sleep deprivation is a bitch! And if you dare complain how exhausted you are feeling, you are sure to get the same old answer: 'You need to do sleep training.'

You don't want unhelpful advice that undermines your confidence and makes you feel as though you are depriving your child for life. But, if you don't want to leave your baby to cry, you are likely to be told, 'You are just postponing the inevitable,' and 'You are making a rod for your back,' or 'You are depriving your baby of an important skill by not teaching him to sleep.'

Sadly, despite what you feel in your heart, these

comments will almost certainly induce feelings of self-doubt and confusion as you feel torn between responding to little night howls and rigid advice that ignores or dismisses the powerful biological connection between you and your baby.

> When my son was waking to feed constantly, I remember feeling that because I wouldn't sleep train him, it somehow meant I wasn't permitted to 'complain' about my exhaustion.
>
> Claire

The pressure to have a baby who self-settles and 'sleeps all night' can create confusion and anxiety even before you welcome your precious child into the world and if you are the sleep-deprived parent of a newborn and are desperately trying to regain some sense of control over your life, it can be tempting to grasp at whatever promises of a good night's sleep are being made, no matter who is offering this advice.

Perhaps now would be a good time to consider that the people who offer rigid advice, like the person who coined the term 'sleeping like a baby', may not actually have a baby at their house. Or, if they do, their child is in the care of a good mother during the wee small hours. Seriously though, there are some important points to bear in mind about people offering rigid advice about infant sleep management. First, it is much easier to ignore infant signalling (and night howls) when the wakeful child isn't hormonally or biologically connected to you. It is also much easier to be 'logical' when you aren't the person who is sleep-deprived. This can also account for how seemingly sensible advice that is totally inappropriate for your baby can leave you feeling undermined – after all, who, in a sleep-deprived state, can come up with a witty, assertive response when they most need one?

When Jair was around six months old, a close friend, James, who was much older than me and my partner – and who had grown children of his own – came to visit us at our home one evening. During his visit, Jair woke and could be heard crying on the baby monitor from where we sat in the dining room. Knowing full well that this person advocated 'crying it out', I sat motionless at the table while Jair became increasingly distressed.

When I was pregnant, this friend had kindly advised us that the only way to ensure our baby wouldn't 'manipulate' us would be to let him cry himself to sleep in his cot for each day and night sleep until he learned to self-soothe. At this point in my parenting journey, I wasn't very confident and I cared what this person thought. (Funny how time and another child makes any care whatsoever completely redundant: a squirt of breast milk across the table may have been a better response to the comments that would follow!) My younger self, however, sat there paralysed with fear. Jair's whimpers had elevated into a fully distressed cry. (Remember, I didn't leave Jair to cry normally so after a few minutes he was desperate to know where I was.)

I slowly rose to my feet and went into the room

to settle Jair on the breast. Once he was asleep, I placed him back in his bed and returned to our guest in the dining room. I had just sat down when Jair had awoken again. I felt my face flush as I tried to avoid eye contact with our guest. Again, I hesitated . . .

Jair's cries elevated but more quickly this time. I knew that I wanted to go to him immediately; to run into his room and scoop him up as I would any other night, but I was being watched (and judged) and I cared way too much what this man thought about us as parents.

After what felt like hours but was only a few minutes, I mustered up the courage and rose to my feet, leaving the table to tend to my baby a second time. Again, I settled him on the breast, placed him in his bed asleep and returned to the dining table. This time I could sense some tension but, thankfully, my husband kept the conversation going. As I studied the embarrassing pile of dust bunnies on the floor next to our guest's feet, I sensed James's eyes settle on me. The sound of a crying baby had broken the conversation for a third time. I met James's gaze and we stared at each other, almost like in one of those Western movies where the villain makes squinted eyes at the hero in some dusty main street of a country town, with weapons drawn and ready for the shoot out. 'Leave him, Dani,' he said. 'Don't you go to him now; you leave him to cry and he'll soon learn . . .'

I've never been one to follow the grain: I delight in being known in my family as the 'Hippie Mum'. My action following Jair's third waking that night revealed *the true destiny of what we had thought was a lifelong friendship with James. Breaking my eyes from his, I got up from the table and went to my baby. I comforted Jair at the breast once more and this time I stayed with him while he slept in my arms contently until our guest left our home, taking with him the unreasonable, inappropriate and disrespectful expectations that he brought with him. As it would happen, the next day, I noticed two cutting teeth in Jair's gums which must have been causing him a great deal of grief the night before . . .*

Dani

Attachment

You may have heard the term accidental parenting. It implies that you, the parents, have inadvertently caused (or will cause) your baby to have sleeping difficulties if you encourage 'bad habits', such as letting your baby fall asleep in your arms or not following a strict regime of one sort or another.

The truth is, there is no accident about how you feel when your baby calms and dozes in your arms, opening heavy eyelids to meet your gaze then perhaps giving a tiny smile before his eyes flutter shut again with delicate lashes resting against little pink cheeks, his warm body snuggled next to your own. Nor is it a sign of weakness or indulgence on your part that you can't resist your baby's cries to be soothed to sleep. Rather, it is due to what scientists call the 'chemistry of attachment'.

This is a massive hormonal upheaval that begins during pregnancy, ensuring that you and your baby are chemically primed to fall in love when you meet each other face-to-face or, rather, skin-to-skin, at birth. It is nature's insurance that your baby will signal for exactly the care she needs to grow and thrive, and that your strong connection with her will help you understand and meet these needs as she adapts to the world outside the womb.

During the last trimester of pregnancy your body brews a cocktail of hormones, and your pituitary gland, which produces this 'mummy margarita', doubles in size and remains enlarged for up to six months postpartum. This means that for as long as six months after your baby is born, your emotional mindset will be irresistibly affected by shifting levels of hormones. This powerful hormonal hangover has such universally intense effects on mothers' inner lives that it is documented by researchers under a variety of labels including 'maternal preoccupation' and 'motherhood mindset'. This more intuitive mindset can be quite at odds with our modern lifestyles and often comes as a shock to women who have previously been in a more goal-oriented and solution-focused space prior to having a baby. Now, it seems that control is out the window and logic has left the building, as the skills that used to keep things neat and tidy (literally) are no longer relevant. This is why the baby instruction manual that advised an efficient program of sleep management seemed so sensible while you were pregnant, but now makes you feel like a failure as neither your baby nor you seem able to slot neatly into the prescribed timetable.

If you can appreciate this new, responsive state as nature's preparation for creating a synchrony between you and the instinctual world of your newborn, you will understand why there is such a struggle between the 'logic' of sleep-training advice and your urge to respond to your baby.

> *I was thinking about what keeps you going in the early days, especially the ability to function on barely any sleep, and I think it's love. The love you feel for your baby, and the need to nurture the little one is what keeps you going and gives you this almost superhuman ability to be patient and gentle and strong through those difficult times. Of course everyone copes differently but I think for me it was the love that really kept me going on an otherwise empty tank. I am so in love with Luna. It is the purest, most all-encompassing, most divine feeling – she is such a delight. When she wakes up and I hear her little voice it means I have to stop whatever it is I'm doing, no matter how important, and see to her. I think, Yay! I get to hold my precious darling again! and I can't wait to go in and pick her up and cuddle her.*
>
> **Alice**

Two of the major players in this magical baby love potion are prolactin, a hormone that promotes milk production and is often referred to as the mothering hormone because of its calming effect that is said to make you more responsive to your baby, and oxytocin, also known as the love hormone. Oxytocin encourages feelings of caring and sensitivity to others and helps us to recognise non-verbal cues more readily. It is released during social contact as well as during love-making, but the release of oxytocin is especially pronounced with skin-to-skin contact. Oxytocin itself is part of a complex hormonal balance. A sudden release creates an urge towards loving that can be directed in different ways depending on the presence of other hormones. For example, with a high level of prolactin, the urge to love is directed towards your baby.

Breastfeeding is a powerful enhancer of the effects of these love hormones, which are released by both mothers and babies, who produce their own oxytocin in response to nursing. However, physical contact with your baby will also stimulate the release of oxytocin, so if you are bottle-feeding you can chemically boost the bond with your baby if you 'bottle nurse' with cuddles and skin contact, rather than prop him up to feed (something you should never do, for safety reasons) or hand him to others.

Bonding with your baby isn't just a mum thing. Recent research suggests that expectant and new fathers actually experience biological and hormonal changes that prepare them for parenting too: in a 2012 study from the University of Notre Dame, Indiana, anthropologist Lee Gettler shows that dads who sleep near their children (on the same sleep surface) experience a drop in testosterone compared to fathers who sleep alone.

Earlier studies by Gettler and others have shown that when men become fathers, especially in the first month after birth, their testosterone decreases, sometimes dramatically, and that those fathers who spend the most time in hands-on care – playing with their children, feeding them or reading to them – have lower testosterone levels again. Authors of these studies speculate that the drop in testosterone is a biological adjustment that helps men shift their priorities when children come along. While high testosterone levels have been linked to aggression, extroversion and risk-taking, drops in testosterone have been linked to fathers' responsiveness to their children. However, just in case you are worried this will affect your manliness or your sex drive, you can relax – it turns out that in one of these studies, partnered fathers were getting more sex than single men without children!

The hormones prolactin and cortisol, both connected with pregnant women, have been shown to rise significantly in men in the three weeks before birth is due. It seems that being near your pregnant partner and the effects of her pheromones trigger hormonal changes in expectant dads. When your baby is born, cuddling and playing with your little one will also elicit the release of prolactin, the hormone of tender nurturing, along with oxytocin, the love hormone, and beta endorphins, the feel-good hormones that are also known as the hormones of pleasure and reward. This means that the more you interact with your baby right from the start, the happier you will feel. In turn you will want to play more, and the better your relationship with your baby will develop. And in case you are worried that playing with your baby will make you less 'manly', the good news is that these lower testosterone levels won't affect your libido – they are still within normal levels. Every nappy you change, every cuddle you share and every game of peekaboo that has you and your baby chuckling with delight is an emotional investment in your baby's wellbeing and his trust in you.

When our first child was born, we lived in a one-bedroom apartment in a block of eight in a dense part of St Kilda. Lots of things were special with the arrival of our first child and we wanted to bring our new son to the apartment as all the other residents had been so much a part of our life for the preceding five years. Nonetheless, living in close proximity to other residents had its own challenges, especially once the novelty of a newborn started to wear off. In particular, the residents downstairs were not as in love with our child as we were. In the middle of the night when our child started to cry we were just as aware of our neighbours as we were of the need to settle our son. Thus began a ritual of taking Tommaso for a walk in the warm summer evenings through the streets of St Kilda.

Our walks could occur at any time from midnight to 3 or even 5 a.m. We went on cold windy nights or on warm nights when there were lots of people still enjoying St Kilda's offerings. Tommaso would always fall asleep within a hundred metres of the apartment and the long walk was really to ensure that he fell into a deep sleep for when we returned back home . . . The cooling sea breezes, the walking and the feeling of being held helped Tommaso sleep comfortably through the night.

In many ways I think it is strange to put a baby into a cot and tell them to sleep – this must feel quite unnatural. Instead, the walking and the feeling of being held must feel far more soothing to a child so small as they adjust to life away from their mother's body. These walks now belong to the mythology of our family as we talk about the days we strolled the streets together in a romantic and special way. Tommaso tells me he remembers the walks. Maybe he does and maybe he doesn't, but the walks did more than settle a crying baby – they became a way to connect father and child in a unique way that was borne out of necessity rather than choice.

Antony

Whichever parent you are – and whether you are an adoptive parent or a same-sex partner – the more you connect with your baby through touch, eye contact, smell and talking, the stronger your connection will be and the more difficult you will find it to ignore your baby's signals. And this is exactly as nature intended.

What's best for baby?

Baby sleep-training advocates seldom consider the baby's experience. A prime example of this is that most research into infant sleep-training methods defines the number of uninterrupted hours babies sleep as the single measure of success, without considering the immediate or longer-term effects on the babies' wellbeing or the parents' sense of competence. Your baby doesn't have an agenda, he isn't trying to manipulate you or to deliberately inconvenience you, he is simply expressing natural biological urges to be nurtured and nourished and to feel safe. He has no control over his needs or how these will be met. Because your baby's wellbeing is your primary responsibility, the possibility that you may have inadvertently caused *any* damage to your relationship with your baby or your baby's sense of trust can be devastating.

> With my youngest, I said I was never going to use controlled crying. One night, after he had been waking every fifteen minutes and I was exhausted, I left him to cry. I wasn't trying to teach him anything, but I just couldn't get up again. I had tried him in bed with me and he crawled all over me and annoyed my husband. After a while, I put him in his cot and just walked out. I was tired and angry and couldn't do it anymore.
>
> Leaving him in his cot was probably the safest thing for him. My husband thought I was starting controlled crying (he thinks it's an okay thing to do and keeps suggesting it), and put ear-plugs in and went back to sleep! I left Billy for about fifteen minutes, who was about ten months old, before I started crying myself. I went and picked him up and he promptly fell asleep in my arms from exhaustion.
>
> The next night he cried as soon as I put him in his cot. Prior to this, he had happily put himself to sleep after a feed, although he would still wake a lot during

*the night. But after I left him to cry, he would only
go in his cot when he was already asleep. I got very
angry at myself after this episode. I think he is over the
trauma of this, but he no longer puts himself to sleep.*

Amy

Like many mothers of older, more active babies, Amy discovered that the notion of snuggling back to sleep with her baby in the parental bed wasn't a solution to his waking, and a lack of support left her little choice but to ensure her baby's safety by leaving him in his cot when she became overwhelmed by exhaustion and frustration.

There are a number of reasons why older babies may wake frequently, from separation anxiety (which peaks at about one year) and 'practising' new mobility skills in their sleep, to discomfort from teething or sensitivity to new foods. Some parents of mobile babies find that they can resettle their babies on a larger, single-bed mattress on the floor (in a childproof space) where the baby has more room to move without disturbing himself or his parents. Others have success putting a cot close to their own bed so they can pat or stroke their baby but he has his own space. However, the middle of the night is not conducive to logical thoughts or clear communication channels between exhausted parents and we should never underestimate how exhaustion can affect our choices, our relationships, or what we may do at any given moment in order to make it through the night.

Cot resistance is not an uncommon reaction in babies over six months who are left to cry. On Amy's part, as this was only a one-off and not a deliberate plan to train her baby by repeatedly ignoring his cries, it seems unfair that she is also burdened with feelings that she may have caused lasting trauma. In fact, I like to reassure parents that if your baby protests strongly at being left to cry, this seems to be a healthy indication that your child will not easily give up on you or abandon signalling for appropriate responses to his needs.

Not guilty

The maternal art of self-flagellation could almost become an Olympic sport, whatever the age of our child. Guilt is pretty much synonymous with being a mother. So please, be gentle on yourself and remember, we can only ever do our best with the information and resources we have available to us at the time, and sometimes in desperation we don't always make the same choices that we might have with different support.

> I'm a midwife and a mother – professional versus maternal – and sometimes the ideas and notions of each role clash. I was very comfortable with each of my babies when they were very little. I didn't have to be taught how to bathe, swaddle, hold or change my baby like a lot of brand-new mums . . . I could do all that with my eyes closed. Another thing that I have spent a lot of nights doing over the last seven years is putting babies to sleep, both at work (I only work night-duty)

and home. My first son fussed with colic and screamed. Then he got clingy and more fussy. So I followed a routine – one thing I was sure of when I had a baby was that he would sleep in his room and we would sleep in our room. So I did the controlled crying thing – no eye contact, walk away from the cot, let him scream, go back to comfort but don't pick him up, leave him longer each time. It went on for hours. When it didn't work after a week or ten days we'd go back to comforting him more and then trying to transfer him to the cot when asleep. Then we'd start all over again . . .

When the second baby came home he went straight into our bed, breastfed on demand (like the first son) and then cuddled up next to mum or dad at night and slept until the next feed. He was a dream baby, and went into a cot at four months, sleeping through the night. But every single night until he was about eighteen months old, he was rocked to sleep in our recliner and then placed into bed.

The third baby was a girl! I came home less than twenty-four hours after the birth, and found we had another fractious baby. We faced almost exactly what we had four years earlier with our first child. She co-slept with us for nearly twelve months, slept in a cot next to our bed for six months, then went into her own bed at eighteen months in the boys' room but still needed someone to lie down with her for a little while before going to sleep. She would hold tightly onto our clothes or hair, just to make sure we weren't moving anywhere.

Do I think that I have permanently damaged my first child beyond belief because I let him cry for hours and hours when he was a baby? No. There were some days when it was safer for me to be standing in the shower crying while he was in the cot doing the same thing.

Do I wish I'd done things differently? Yes. I wish I had been less rigid, and had gone with my gut feelings rather than trying to do things by the book and to routine.

Cheryl

If you have already given controlled crying a try, my intention is not to make you feel guilty but to help you make informed choices, whatever you decide is best for your family right now. And when I talk about leaving babies to cry I am referring to distressed crying, not the wind-down grizzling of a tired baby. However, I believe it is best to hold a crying baby or child whatever the reasons (don't you like a hug when you feel fragile and teary?). As a responsive parent you will know the difference between your baby's signals and their urgency and how best to respond. If you aren't quite sure yet, see the section about reading your baby's cues.

Until Bella was about six weeks old I was pretty depressed. During this time I felt incredibly guilty about a lot of things. I felt bad that I hadn't formed an immediate bond with her. I felt bad that I couldn't breastfeed. I felt bad that she wasn't sleeping as long as other babies. I felt guilty that I wasn't a supermum and that I wasn't enjoying being a mother as much as

I thought I would. The list goes on. After talking with other mums I was amazed that so many others experienced feelings similar to mine in the first couple of months. I just wish that my friends and I had been honest in the beginning so we could have offered support to one another. I took so much comfort in knowing that I wasn't alone.

Leah

The 'science' of sleep training

It is easy to feel confused about which is the sensible way to rear our children when there is dissent among childcare experts. As you can see from the quotes below, conflicting advice about infant sleep is not new. For many years we have had what I like to call the 'tamers', who advocate training infants to self-soothe, and the 'cuddlers', who encourage parents to respond and comfort their wakeful infants.

The cries of an infant are the voice of Nature, supplicating relief. It can express its wants in no other language.

Mrs Parkes, *Domestic Duties*, 1825

If, by the second week, they are left to go to sleep in their cots, and allowed to find out that they do not get their way by crying, they at once become reconciled.

John Walsh, *Manual of Domestic Economy*, 1850s

Methods of training babies to self-soothe and sleep alone have become somewhat more sophisticated than simply leaving babies to cry it out, and these days leaving a baby to cry has a label: 'extinction'. This is based on the behavioural principle that if parents don't respond when their baby or young child cries, the rewarding effects of this attention will be removed, and the undesirable behaviour (the crying) will be extinguished. In all fairness to the professionals who devised practices such as controlled crying, their intention was undoubtedly to introduce a more humane approach to baby training. Hence, the academic term for the alternative approach (to extinction) of checking on babies and offering reassurance at predetermined intervals is 'graduated extinction'.

When controlled crying or graduated extinction was first advocated around thirty years ago, it was recommended for infants over six months old, not newborns. While there are still professionals who feel comfortable with variations of controlled crying for older babies (some advice is less extreme than other versions), many of these people would see any such methods as inappropriate for younger babies. However, in other cases, the thin edge of the wedge has slipped: popular advice by various authors and even some health professionals now commonly includes leaving babies as young as a few weeks old to cry in order to teach them to sleep, much like the advice offered in the 1850s. Some modern sleep-training methods are euphemistically labelled 'controlled comforting', 'controlled soothing', 'spaced soothing', 'gradual withdrawal' or 'pick up put down' and within each definition there can be different recommendations about how long to leave babies to cry and how often or how long to comfort. Others simply advise leaving the baby to cry until it falls asleep.

In an article in the *New York Times*, 'Sleep Training at 8 Weeks: Do You Have the Guts?' writer and new mother Aimee Molloy describes how, at her baby's eight-week paediatric checkup, she was advised to sleep train. As she proudly told her doctor how well her baby was breast-feeding and gaining weight, and that she was sleeping six- to eight-hour stretches already, her paediatrician told Aimee that the baby could be sleeping twelve hours at night. The doctor then advised putting the baby in her cot at 7 p.m., closing the door and returning at 7 a.m. Of course she would cry but after about three nights the crying would stop when the baby realised nobody was coming to her rescue.

Although many baby sleep trainers and even some health professionals claim there is no proof of harm from practices such as controlled crying or, as in Aimee's case, the 'cry it out' method, it is worth noting that there is a vast difference between 'no proof of harm' and 'proof of no harm'. In fact, a growing number of health profes-sionals are now claiming that training infants to sleep too deeply, too soon, is not in babies' best psychological or physiological interests. A policy statement on controlled crying issued by the Australian Association of Infant Mental Health (AAIMHI) advises, 'Controlled crying is not consistent with what infants need for their optimal emotional and psychological health, and may have unin-tended negative consequences.'

Needing a published study to tell us a baby (or anyone, for that matter) will be distressed if we shut him in a room alone and don't respond to his cries is like needing research to tell us the grass will grow if it rains. Even basic commonsense tells us that a baby left alone for twelve hours could aspirate vomit and choke, or become overheated from crying (a SIDS risk). Or, if she has 'got the picture' that nobody is coming to her rescue, she may not signal at all, even if she is in trouble. While there is certainly a difference in physical safety between checking on a crying baby and shutting the door overnight, there are no published studies telling us how long it is 'safe' to leave a baby to cry, if at all. Moreover, there is evidence that there is potential harm in neglecting babies' needs in order to train them to sleep.

Babies who are forced to sleep alone (or cry, because many do not sleep) for hours may miss out on both adequate nutrition and sensory stimulation such as touch, which is as important as food for infant development. Leaving a baby to cry it out in order to enforce a strict routine when the baby may, in fact, be hungry, is similar to expecting an adult to adopt a strenuous exercise program accompanied by a reduced food intake. The result of expending energy through crying while being deprived of food is likely to be weight loss and failure to thrive.

Paediatrician William Sears has claimed that 'babies who are "trained" not to express their needs may appear to be docile, compliant or "good" babies. Yet, these babies could be depressed babies who are shutting down the expression of their needs.' Babies can indeed be 'brand-new and blue' with an actual diagnosis of clinical depression. Often the predisposing conditions for depression in infants are beyond our control, such as trauma due to early hospitalisation and medical treatments. However, if we consider the baby's perspective, it is easy to understand how extremely rigid regimes can also be associated with infant depression and why it isn't worth risking, especially if your child has already experienced early separation. You too would withdraw and become sad if the people you loved avoided eye contact, as some sleep-training techniques advise, and repeatedly ignored your cries.

Leaving a baby to cry evokes physiological responses that increase stress hormones. Crying infants experience an increase in heart rate, body temperature and blood pressure. These reactions are likely to result in overheating and, along with vomiting due to extreme distress, could pose a potential risk of SIDS in vulnerable infants.

There may also be longer-term emotional effects.

Infancy is a time of rapid development; a time when tiny brains are being wired. Babies need our help to learn how to regulate their emotions, meaning that when we respond to and soothe their cries, we help them understand that when they are upset, they can calm down. On the other hand, when infants are left alone to cry it out, they fail to develop the understanding that they can regulate their own emotions. Responsive nurturing encourages the development of parts of the brain that regulate emotions. A longitudinal study of depressed and healthy preschool children who underwent neuroimaging at school age showed that children who experienced responsive early nurturing had a larger hippocampal volume – a brain region that is key to memory and stress modulation. This means that by responding to your baby when she is young, when she is older she will have a better capacity to soothe herself and calm down if she is feeling upset, angry or anxious.

The development of healthy biological and chemical responses, which will support future mental health, is another aspect of early brain wiring that may be affected by ignoring babies' signals. In early childhood, cortisol receptors are developing in the brain and the more cortisol receptors, the better your baby's capacity to mop up stress in the future as the stress hormone cortisol is released. Moreover, night-time breastmilk is rich in tryptophan, a precursor to serotonin. Serotonin receptors affect neurotransmitters and hormones that influence various biological and neurological processes such as aggression, anxiety, appetite, cognition, learning, memory, mood, nausea and sleep. This could mean that night feeds (if an individual baby needs them – some babies choose to drop night feeds at early ages) may play an important role in development of serotonin receptors and future wellbeing.

There is compelling evidence that increased levels of stress hormones may cause permanent changes in the stress responses of the infant's developing brain. These changes then affect memory, attention and emotion, and can trigger an elevated response to stress throughout life, including a predisposition to later anxiety and depressive disorders. English psychotherapist Sue Gerhardt, author of *Why Love Matters: How Affection Shapes a Baby's Brain*, explains that when a baby is upset, the hypothalamus produces cortisol. In normal amounts cortisol is fine, but if a baby is exposed for too long or too often to stressful situations (such as being left to cry) its brain becomes flooded with cortisol. Too much cortisol is linked to depression and fearfulness; too little to emotional detachment and aggression.

A study by Wendy Middlemiss at the University of North Texas affirms that babies release cortisol in large amounts when they are left to cry during sleep training. They are still releasing the cortisol even after sleep training has 'worked' (that is, even after the baby has stopped crying and is sleeping). Studying babies aged four to ten months, Middlemiss and her team monitored the levels of cortisol as they were left to fall asleep without comfort from a carer. Researchers measured the length of time they cried over successive nights as their mothers waited in a nearby room. Mothers' cortisol levels were also measured.

By the third night, although the babies cried less, their cortisol levels remained elevated. This means that although sleep training achieved a sleeping baby, the babies were still distressed. Initially, the mothers' cortisol levels were elevated and matched their babies' levels while the babies were crying. However, as the babies' crying reduced and they slept, the mothers' cortisol levels decreased. This disassociation between the babies' behavioral and physiological responses means that although the babies were still distressed, the mothers were no longer in synchrony with their babies. The babies were distressed but because they were no longer signalling that they needed help, their mothers weren't attuned to their needs.

Stress levels in infancy may have implications for learning, too. While it seems fairly obvious that a calm baby will be available for learning, studies have shown that children with the lowest scores on mental and motor ability tests were those with the highest cortisol levels in their blood. There is also research showing that children with anxiety disorders have a higher level of sleep difficulties as infants. Although these studies weren't about controlled crying and I am making no direct connection, my point is that perhaps some of the babies who are presenting with sleep difficulties are infants who need extra help to regulate their emotions or are more sensitive to stress, so it is possible that these little people would be more at risk if they were exposed to controlled crying.

Our first baby was fairly easygoing, we had a bit of trouble getting her to sleep when she was tiny, I think because we didn't realise how much sleep babies need or how quickly they get overtired, but it wasn't too much of a drama and she slept well at night, which made life much easier. She did wake at night (as you would completely expect), but quickly settled after a feed. At nine months, after I had returned to work, we did controlled crying for two nights. It was so tough, but on night three and thereafter, she slept through and we thought, gee that was good.

Our second baby was a challenging baby from the get-go, very spewy (turned out he had reflux) and he rarely slept. We had feeding issues due to a problem with one of my breasts and I had to mix feed from eight weeks. But the biggest problem really was the lack of sleep. He would wake six to eight times a night, and was nearly impossible to comfort or get to sleep – day or night.

After three months of hell we had a maternal and child health nurse come out to help settle him and give us some advice. Even she couldn't get him to sleep! By six months things were worse than ever and we were absolutely wrecked. In desperation we sought assistance from a sleep consultant (locally referred to as the Sleep Witch). She would come out to your home, spend the night with you and would then call daily for a couple of weeks to coach you and follow up. The premise was that your child would sleep through within three nights.

We saw minimal improvement, but she assured us that we were making progress and he'd soon be sleeping. So we kept at it, and at it . . . My alarm bells should have been clanging by now, but in desperation and feeling like we had tried everything else and failed, we kept going and going and going. We had previously tried a soothing CD, white noise, light on, light off, sitting next to the cot, co-sleeping, an osteopath and more – so many things!

I now realise that we let expectations and what everyone else's babies were doing make us feel like we were failing. We didn't have support from family or friends (they live hours away) and that left us exhaust-ed, defeated and willing to do anything. But I had no idea to what extent the lack of sleep would affect my *gorgeous golden-haired boy. Now, at six years old, he is suffering anxiety and OCD-like symptoms and has behavioural issues. He's not able to concentrate at school unless he's got one-on-one attention. He doesn't cope at all if he feels we are going somewhere without him or if he is being rushed. In these situations he says over and over, 'Don't leave me!' It's really difficult to live like this, but more so, to see him live like this. We are currently waiting to have him assessed by a series of medical professionals who will hopefully equip us with the skills and coping mechanisms to help our son. His behaviour affects the whole family, particularly his siblings, but also me and my husband. It's stressful, embarrassing and difficult not to react to his behaviour. But most of all, it's heartbreaking! We honestly believe, and our doctor agrees, that sleep training and the duration of our attempts play a significant part in his temperament and behaviour. It's awful to hear that, to admit it and know it was our choice to do it. I feel as though I have let my son down and I second-guess myself whenever I question why it worked so easily for our daughter – were we just lucky? Or did she simply give up trying to get our attention?*

Alice

For mothers like Alice, whose baby may have been more vulnerable or who may have had underlying issues that weren't addressed, the guilt and self-doubt associated with her parenting decisions are devastatingly cruel. She was simply following the advice of professionals under extremely difficult circumstances. The thing is, we don't know which babies are more vulnerable or which ones may be at risk from being left to cry to sleep. Or when evidence of harm will surface – or which parts of our parenting could have caused harm. Although it is natural to blame ourselves whenever our children are hurting, we don't need the second-guessing or guilt or regret – that awful feeling of 'if only' when this happens. This is why I advise parents to filter any advice they feel unsure of by asking, 'Is it safe? Is it respectful? Does it feel right?' And, if at any time what you are doing feels stressful to you or your baby, no matter who has given you this advice, ditch it or seek another opinion.

One of the arguments for using controlled crying is that it works, but perhaps the definition of success needs to be examined more closely. In the small number of studies undertaken, while most babies will indeed stop waking when they are left to cry, success varies from an extra hour's sleep each night to little difference between babies who underwent sleep training and those who didn't, eight weeks later. In one Australian study of controlled crying in infants over six months, just over 30 per cent of parents said it didn't work. In a Canadian study, 48 per cent of parents had tried sleep training four or more times (before and after six months) but regardless of how many times they had started sleep training only 14 per cent of parents said it eliminated night-wakings whereas 42 per cent of parents said it did not reduce night-wakings at all.

To me, this suggests that even if harsher regimes work initially, babies are likely to start waking again as they reach new developmental stages or if they get sick, otherwise why would parents repeat the process so many times? If night-waking is a problem for parents (if it doesn't bother you, it isn't a problem) then this is a sign that your baby needs comfort for some reason and if we simply extinguish the crying by ignoring it, the night-waking will persist as long as the underlying issues are not attended to.

> *Chloe has always been a good sleeper, but I believe that part of the reason for that is because we have never tried to impose what we think she should do on her (sleep in her own bed if she wants to, sleep in our bed, or sleep in a cot if she wants to, sleep in a sling or hammock etc). We have found that when she is good and ready, she does these things by herself without us putting pressure on her. For example, she stopped sleeping in a sling because she grew and it became too uncomfortable for her. She no longer likes to sleep in our bed because she has grown again and with three of us in the bed, it is now getting too uncomfortable for her so she prefers her cot . . . Her emotional need to be close to us has never been threatened so she is comfortable moving onto the next stage when she is physically ready.*
>
> Liz

> *I am so glad that I didn't cave and do controlled crying. My baby is now fifteen months old and even my husband has thanked me for standing my ground on this one. Learning to listen to what is in my heart when it*

comes to parenting has been the greatest gift.
I know myself better now and I think it has helped me
in every area of my life. Just knowing that my instinc-
tive responses are the right ones gives me so much
confidence as a mother.

Michelle

Controlled crying and other similar regimes may indeed work to produce a self-soothing, solitary sleeping infant. However, the trade-off could be an anxious, clingy or hyper-vigilant child or even worse, a child whose trust is broken. Unfortunately, we can't measure attributes such as trust and empathy, which are the basic skills for forming all relationships. We can't, for instance, give a child a trust quotient like we can give him an intelligence quotient. One of the saddest emails I have received was from a mother who did controlled crying with her one-year-old toddler.

After a week of controlled crying he slept, but he
stopped talking (he was saying single words). For the
past year, he has refused all physical contact from
me. If he hurts himself, he goes to his older brother (a
preschooler) for comfort. I feel devastated that I have
betrayed my child.

Sonia

It is the very principle that makes controlled crying work that is of greatest concern: when controlled crying 'succeeds' in teaching a baby to fall asleep alone, it is due to a process that neurobiologist Bruce Perry calls the 'defeat response'. Normally, when humans feel threatened, our bodies flood with stress hormones and we go into fight-or-flight mode. But there is a third survival response. Babies can't fight and they can't flee, so they communicate their distress by crying. When infant cries are ignored, this trauma elicits a 'freeze' or 'defeat' response. As we saw in the studies by Wendy Middlemiss, babies eventually abandon their crying even though the baby's brain is flooded with stress hormones. Paediatrician William Sears calls this the 'shut down syndrome' – the baby's nervous system shuts down the emotional pain and the striving to reach out. This is a basic survival mechanism to preserve homeostasis and not a sign that you have taught a baby to sleep.

One explanation for the success of 'crying it out' is that when an infant's defeat response is triggered often enough, the child will become habituated to this. That is, each time the child is left to cry, he 'switches' more quickly to this response. This is why babies may cry for say, an hour the first night, twenty minutes the following night and fall asleep almost immediately on the third night (if you are 'lucky'). They are 'switching off' (and sleeping) more quickly, not learning a legitimate skill.

Whether sleep 'success' is due to behavioural principles (that is, a lack of 'rewards' when baby wakes) or whether the baby is overwhelmed by a stress reaction, the saddest risk of all is that as he tries to communicate in the only way available to him, the baby who is left to cry in order to teach him to sleep will learn a much crueller lesson – that he cannot make a difference, so what is the point of reaching out. This is learned helplessness.

There is good news for parents who can't bear to train their baby to sleep by leaving them to cry: neuroscientists and clinicians have documented that loving interactions that are sensitive to a child's needs influence the way the brain grows and can increase the number of connections between nerve cells. The AAIMH advises: 'Infants are more likely to form secure attachments when their distress is responded to promptly, consistently and appropriately. Secure attachments in infancy are the foundation for good adult mental health.'

So, when you adopt the perspective that your baby's night howls are the expression of a need, that she is not trying to 'manipulate' you, and you respond appropriately according to her age and needs, you are not only making her smarter, but you will be hardwiring her brain for future mental health.

Where is the manual?

'I would be ashamed to admit to the Indians that where I come from the women do not feel themselves capable of raising children until they have read the instructions written by a strange man.'

Jean Leidloff, *The Continuum Concept*

As you gaze lovingly at the tiny bundle in your arms, you probably feel equally protective and confused. Are you asking yourself, 'What are we doing? Why didn't she come with a manual?'

To borrow a phrase from Canadian psychologist Jan Hunt, 'your baby is the book'. By spending time with your baby, watching her movements and her facial expressions, you will begin to understand her patterns of behaviour and learn to read her non-verbal language so that you can respond accordingly. When this happens, it will feel as though you have discovered a key that lets you enter her world: you won't find yourself hovering over the cot trying to make your baby sleep when she isn't ready to; avoiding social events because you don't know whether they will fit your baby's sleep patterns; or find yourself trying to poke food into her tiny mouth when she would be happier playing with you. Instead, by observing your baby's behaviour and learning to read her cues, you will be able to respond sensitively and with respect to your baby at specific times and you will be able to create a gentle rhythm to the day that suits you both without unnecessary struggles. (See Baby's day, page 205.)

Sleep cycles

Although you will intuitively become aware of your baby's nuances and moods, it can help to understand that her behaviour does follow the pattern of a typical baby. For instance, you will notice that your baby moves through varying states of consciousness from sleeping to waking and in between. Psychologists have labelled six states of consciousness that you will come to recognise. As well as active sleep and quiet sleep, there are three awake states – quiet alert, active alert and crying. The final state is drowsiness, as your baby transitions between sleep and wakefulness or vice-versa.

Quiet sleep

If you watch your baby as he sleeps, you will see him move through sleep cycles. When he is in a quiet sleep state, he will lie still and his face will be relaxed with no eye movements. Although he may startle or twitch occasionally, in a quiet sleep state, your baby's body will be still and his breathing will be regular. This is not a good time to try to offer a feed, for instance, as your baby will probably not cooperate.

Active sleep

In an active or lighter sleep state, as the label implies, your baby will be more active and his breathing less regular – it may be slightly faster than it is in quiet sleep. Your baby may move his arms and legs or stir his entire body, and in active sleep babies often grimace or give tiny grins or frowns and you may notice your baby's eyelids flutter or see his eyes moving beneath his eyelids. Sometimes during active sleep, babies make sucking movements and may even make brief crying noises without waking. If you wait a few moments and watch, rather than pick him up or offer a feed, your baby may go back into a deeper sleep.

This can be a helpful tactic to remember during the night, so that you give your baby an opportunity to extend his sleep times when he is ready. Of course if he really needs attention or a feed, he will let you know by waking fully and giving you clear signals!

Drowsiness

Often your baby will arouse into a drowsy state before he wakes fully and, of course, he will become drowsy as he is about to fall asleep. His body movements will be smooth, but he may have some mild startles and his eyelids will look heavy as they open and close over his dull, glazed-looking eyes.

You can pop your baby down to sleep while he is drowsy and he may fall asleep without any help such as rocking or cuddling. If he is drowsy but possibly wakening after a sleep, wait and see if he wakes fully or, if you want to encourage him to wake, perhaps because he has slept a long stretch between daytime feeds, or you want to get ready to go out, very gently offer your baby something to see, hear or suck.

Quiet alert

When your baby is in a quiet alert state, he will pay attention to you rather like a friend who is listening closely to you during a conversation – his eyes will widen and become bright, he will often look directly at your face and eyes and perhaps make little cooing noises. At this time, your baby's movements are generally smooth and coordinated although very young babies can also startle or have jerky movements. These erratic movements are simply due to your baby's immature nervous system, not a sign that you have frightened him or upset him in any way.

In a quiet alert state, your little one will be in a lovely mood for quiet play and learning. He will be able to focus on stimuli such as your voice or a toy as you show it to him. You can encourage this alertness by unwrapping your baby or at least uncovering his hands and arms and placing him in an upright position facing you. Talk gently to him, taking turns at talking and listening by pausing and allowing spaces in the conversation for him to talk back to you. This is also an appropriate time to do an activity such as baby massage (see page 232).

Active alert

In an active alert state your baby's eyes will be open but not as bright and they will dart around. She will make lots of body movements and little noises and may fuss a bit, indicating that she needs a change of pace. This is a great time to engage in play. However, in an active alert state your baby will be more sensitive to noise and hunger. If she has difficulty moving from this active state and becomes fussy, you may need to slow down and stop playing (or remove her from bright lights and noise – such as the sensory stimulation of a shopping centre) before she becomes overstimulated and overwrought.

Crying

Crying is a form of communication, not a sign of manipulation. Your baby is telling you that he needs something or somebody to help soothe him. There are lots of reasons why babies cry, from tiredness, boredom or hunger to discomfort and overstimulation. As you get to know your baby, you will learn his pre-cry signals and by responding to these you may be able to avert a full-blown crying state.

Some babies, especially in the early weeks, cry because they have difficulty moving smoothly between the states described above. At times, your baby may cry simply to release tension, especially if he is overtired. Remember, your child will feel safe if you hold him as he cries: there is a big difference between allowing your baby to cry as a stress release, and leaving him alone to cry it out.

What is my baby saying?

Cues are your baby's way of trying to tell you what she needs. Although it may take a few weeks to get to know your baby's cues, or non-verbal language, if you do some baby-watching, you will be amazed at how even very young babies can give clear signals that they want to interact, would prefer to be given a break from play, or are tired or hungry.

Responding to your baby's cues (day and night) will help your baby develop a sense of trust in his ability to influence his environment and will help him form a secure attachment to you. These are important prerequisites for later emotional development and relationships. Your responsiveness will also help your baby learn what psychologists call 'emotional regulation', which is the capacity to understand that we have control over our emotions. As you soothe your baby, you are teaching him that when he is upset, he can calm down. When babies' signals are ignored, and they escalate to cries that are not responded to, the baby fails to develop the understanding that he can regulate his own emotions.

I'm hungry
Babies give a lot of subtle cues that they are ready to feed, long before they begin to cry – from rooting with their

mouths to making sucking noises and trying to suck on their fists, as well as little noises that say, 'I'm working up to a cry.' If these signals are ignored, they will yell. Crying is a late hunger cue and when we repeatedly wait until a young baby cries (sometimes it is unavoidable), perhaps because we are trying to implement a strict feeding schedule, we can set ourselves on a path to unnecessary feeding problems. (See Feed me, page 154.) Notice where your baby's tongue is when she is yelling – a baby can't latch on to feed when her tongue is up against the roof of her mouth, and if you do manage to calm her enough to latch on and feed, her suck is likely to be disorganised, or she may be exhausted from crying and only take a small feed before falling asleep. This, of course, means that she will probably sleep for a very short time then wake for another feed as her tiny tummy quickly empties.

At night-time, it may take you longer to arouse from your own sleep to respond to your baby's signals before he actually cries but he will usually give a few small warning calls before he works up to distressed wailing. If your baby sleeps near you in the early months you will be surprised how intuitively you will respond to his movements and noises, even if they aren't very loud.

> I have three sons: seven, five and fourteen weeks. With my first two I did the routine, scheduled feeding and looking back now I regret not listening to my heart. I now feed when my son wants to. He sleeps more in our bed than in his cot, which is in our room. The nights he sleeps next to me I get more sleep as I can easily

*comfort him with a cuddle or a breast rather than
getting up out of the bed. My husband is supportive
of the sleeping arrangement . . . we feel it's his right
to sleep near us and be close to us as much as possible.
I feel that having the older children makes us realise
how quickly they grow too.*

Jo

Play with me

Tiny babies have very short periods where they can actually engage and interact with you, but as she grows, your little one will be able to play for longer periods and her signals will become much clearer. When your baby wants you to play, her eyes will become wide and bright and she may purse her tiny lips as though she is saying 'ooh' as she turns towards your voice or looks at your face. Movements of her arms and legs will be smooth (as opposed to jerky) as she reaches out to you – she might grasp your finger or hold onto you. If you respond, your baby will make eye contact and smile, coo, babble or talk. These signals or 'engagement cues' are your baby's way of saying, 'Please play with me.'

Give me a break

When your baby needs a break from what she is doing, she will give very clear 'disengaging' signals such as look-ing away (little babies can only maintain eye contact for short periods so may look away then continue gazing at you after a break) or turning her head away, squirming or kicking, coughing, spitting up or arching her back. Some babies will even put up their hand in a sort of stop sign. More subtle cues that your baby is tiring from playing or needs a change of pace or even activity may be yawning, wrinkling her forehead, frowning or hiccuping. If you keep playing when your baby tries to tell you she wants to stop, she will become agitated and make thrashing movements, or she will start fussing and crying.

I'm sleepy

None of us like being kept awake when we are craving sleep so rather than waiting until your baby is past it, put her to bed as soon as she shows sleepy signs, such as becoming quiet, losing interest in people and toys, making jerky movements (in small babies) or becoming very still (these babies relax and fall asleep easily), yawning, frowning or knotting her eyebrows, clenching her fists into tight balls, rubbing her eyes and ears and fussing. If you miss this window of opportunity, your baby is likely to become grumpy and find it difficult to settle. If you miss your baby's tired signs, she may become hyped up and will be much harder to settle.

> *Barclay always rubs his eyes when he's getting tired and he gets a bit whingy and won't be placated. If he cries to be picked up and then squirms to get down, and doesn't want to feed, then I know he needs sleep!*
>
> **Zoe**

> *Mackenzie didn't really have a sleep routine until she was nine months old. Before this, I just cuddled her*

when she was showing tired signs and then popped her into her cot. She would sleep for about forty minutes, four or five times a day, even if we were out. When she hit nine months everything changed. She only wanted two sleeps and slept anywhere between one to two-and-a-half hours. I now say, 'time for bed', and give her a dummy and she waits at the bottom of the stairs for me to take her up. Being a first-time mum it took me a while to pick up that three hours of wake time just about pulls her up and her mood changes so I know it's time for a sleep!

Andrea

Although these cues are typical signs that most babies use to elicit the care they need, individual babies will not use all of these cues all of the time. Each baby will develop his own mix of signals. For instance, one tired baby may lie still and watch her tiny fist as she becomes increasingly drowsy, another may have less control over his movements which could be jerky if he is young, or seemingly uncoordinated if he is already mobile, and yet another baby may rub his eyes and fuss.

As you play with your baby you will notice a mixture of engagement and disengagement signals, so take your time getting to know your baby's way of communicating when she is enjoying playing, when she is feeling a bit overwhelmed and needs a break, and when she is becoming hungry or tired. Your baby's signals may seem unclear but by spending lots of time just watching your baby and being present with her, along with some trial and error working out what your baby is telling you, you will soon become attuned to each other. She will develop her own unique way of communicating with each person in her world and you and your partner will learn to respond in just the way that suits your baby.

Put yourself in their place

It is easy to simply 'do' things to small children and babies, without considering how intrusive or disrespectful it might feel to them. Just for a moment, put yourself in your baby's bootees: what if you were working on a task (play is a child's work) and somebody scooped you up and began removing your clothes without so much as a please or thank you? And if they then popped you into bed and walked out of the room, expecting you to go to sleep without a fuss?

Empathy is about putting yourself in your baby's place and seeing things from her perspective. Imagine your reaction if you were reading in bed and your partner turned off the light without warning? We can all be mindful how we do things to babies and small children. First, you can tell your baby or toddler what you are about to do, rather than just sneaking up on him. If you want to do something with your baby that isn't absolutely necessary (of course, changing a nappy isn't optional), such as giving him a massage, ask his consent first. You might be wondering what the point is of asking consent from a baby who can't understand you but, as I have discussed, even a tiny baby will be able to give you clear signals that she wants to play, or be picked up, or that she would prefer to be left alone. By responding sensitively to your baby's cues, you are teaching her to say yes and no to things that are pleasurable or not.

How does your baby sleep?

Just like us, each baby is unique and needs a different amount of sleep. Even within the same family, we can have 'high energy' or 'low sleep requirement' children and we can have those who need more sleep. An extreme example of this is one of my own children, who gave up all daytime sleeps at six months old and, contrary to any infant sleep requirement chart I have ever seen, only needed eight hours' sleep in any twenty-four hour period. As I wondered where this baby had stashed the jet fuel he seemed to be snacking on when I wasn't looking (I would have taken some myself if I could have figured out what made him buzz!), I was in shock that my afternoon quiet times had been cut short so prematurely. My then two-year-old was still having a two-hour afternoon nap each day, as well as a good sleep every night. It was hard for me to accept that I could no longer smugly attribute my older child's easy sleep patterns to good management on my part.

Despite advice that my active baby would not grow because, according to my critics, 'Babies grow when they are asleep,' my jet-fuelled baby's height and weight were on the ninetieth percentile. And he crawled and climbed and walked before most other babies his age. (Well, he was awake and practising much harder than his peers!) I was also warned that my baby would be grumpy without sleep. Instead, people would comment on how happy and sociable he was – he still is. As a tall, strong adult, people are now in awe of my son's energy and drive. To this day he needs less sleep than most people I have ever met.

While most babies fit somewhere along a spectrum of normal sleep requirements it can help to realise that whatever chart is used and whatever the average is, there will be babies on either end of the spectrum. According to Australian GP and infant sleep researcher Dr Pamela Douglas, your baby's sleep needs will depend partly on her developmental maturity at birth, which varies significantly between normal babies, and partly on genetic predisposition. She says a newborn may sleep for a total of nine to twenty hours a day, and the whole range is normal. By six months of age, babies can sleep from anywhere between less than nine hours to up to seventeen hours a day. So, like my own second child, your baby could sleep half as much as some other babies the same age and this be perfectly normal. Just as there will be babies with higher and lower sleep needs, babies can vary in the amount of sleep they need on different days. If they have had a busy day practising a new skill or being out and about in stimulating surroundings, they may not sleep much, but the next day they may take longer naps to catch up.

Most infant sleep charts were compiled many years ago when breastfeeding rates were at their lowest, so these observations were based on mostly formula-fed babies, sleeping in rooms by themselves under laboratory study conditions. At this time formula was more difficult to digest so these babies generally did sleep longer than breastfed babies at an earlier age. However, if you are thinking that a bottle of formula and banishment to the nursery may be the answer to your baby's (and your own) sleepless nights, you could be mistaken. Recent research has found that mothers who breastfeed in the evening actually get an average of forty-five minutes more sleep than those who give formula. This could be due to the composition of night-time breastmilk: evening breastmilk is rich in tryptophan, a sleep inducing amino acid that is precursor to serotonin. Serotonin is a vital hormone for brain function and development that makes the brain work better, keeps one in a good mood, and helps with sleep cycles. We now know that ingestion of tryptophan in infancy leads to more serotonin receptor development, creating the potential for life-long wellbeing. Night-time breastmilk also has amino acids that promote serotonin synthesis, so evening and night-time breastfeeds could be more important to your baby's development than simply promoting sound sleep.

A 2015 study reported in the *Academy of Breastfeeding Medicine* journal found that night-wakings or night feeds didn't differ between mothers who breastfed or formula fed. In the study, 715 mothers with an infant six to twelve months of age reported their infants' typical night-wakings and feeds alongside any breastfeeding and solid meals. Of infants in this age range, 79 per cent still regularly woke at least once a night, with 61 per cent receiving one or more milk feeds. However, babies who fed more during the day woke less due to hunger overnight. This is not a reason to introduce early solid foods (see Feed me, page 154), but it can be helpful to limit distractions that may reduce feeds during the day. It is also a good reason not to stretch out daytime feeds according to a rigid schedule – consider if your baby needs a certain amount of food in a twenty-four-hour period. If you limit feeds during the day, he will wake at night to get his 'quota'.

Also, please consider the accompanying risks of premature weaning: you could find the trade-off being hours pacing the floor with an unwell baby. And, as you will see later, young babies are much safer sleeping near their parents. Since no parent would knowingly trade their baby's wellbeing for an uninterrupted night's sleep, it is better to measure normal by what is safe and healthy.

It is pointless to waste precious energy by becoming stressed that you don't have a textbook baby. It may be a relief (or not!) to discover that 'all night' in infant sleep studies is defined as five hours and that night howls are more normal than exceptional. According to long-term research at Bristol University (the Avon Longitudinal Study of Parents and Children), at six to eight months only 16 per cent of babies were sleeping straight through, over half woke occasionally, 9 per cent did so on most nights, and 17 per cent woke more than once every night (between two and nine times!).

An Australian study that looked at more than 3000 Queensland children in the first months after birth found that nearly all the babies woke at least once each night, with more than 5 per cent waking at least five times. At three months, two-thirds of the babies were still waking regularly but at four months, half of the babies were sleeping through (remember in infant sleep studies, all night means five hours). However, a very large percentage of babies in the study began waking again, with just under two-thirds regularly waking between ten and twelve months. At this time, 12.5 per cent were waking three or more times a night.

Of course, simply knowing that you are not alone pacing the floor in the wee small hours will not solve your sleep problem. However, understanding the wide range of normal infant sleep can allay fears that you have somehow unwittingly created sleep problems or that you have a particularly difficult baby.

Sleeping like a baby

'Sleeping like a baby' is quite different from adult sleep. Like us, babies' sleep is divided into light (REM or rapid eye movement) sleep and deep (non-REM) sleep. While adults have several levels of deep sleep in comparison to babies, researchers classify newborn sleep as either active or quiet sleep.

If you do some baby watching, you will notice that the label active sleep is very appropriate: you may notice your baby's eyes dart from side to side under his eyelids, he may frown or wriggle his arms and legs, his breathing is irregular and he may even cry or whimper – all without waking. In contrast, during quiet sleep, although your baby may have an occasional startle response or make sucking movements with his mouth, he is generally very still with quiet, regular breathing.

The greatest difference between infant and adult sleep is that newborns and adults have different sleep cycles. While adults have a ninety-minute sleep cycle and spend about 75 per cent of their sleep time in quiet (non-REM) sleep and about 25 per cent in active (or REM) sleep, babies have much shorter sleep cycles of about forty-five minutes and spend twice as much time in active sleep than an adult. Your baby's sleep cycle will be divided into about twenty to twenty-five minutes each of active and deep sleep, and for the first three to four months, she will enter deep sleep through an active sleep state. This is why newborns usually need help to fall asleep – it's not easy to reach a deep sleep when your tiny brain is active and your body is having difficulty being still. Babies also arouse frequently. Arousals are related to the maturity of your baby – the younger the baby, the more arousals are normal. Premature babies, for instance, tend to spend more time in active sleep and may wake more frequently at night than full-term babies for the first few months or even longer. Then again, some premature babies sleep a lot and need to be woken to feed, at least in the early weeks.

According to researchers such as Professor James McKenna, these frequent arousals that are characteristic of infant sleep are part of an infant's inbuilt survival mechanism and may play a protective role against SIDS. Babies need to arouse if there is a breathing obstruction, if they are too hot or too cold (both SIDS risk factors) and of course, in the early weeks at least, babies also need to arouse and breastfeed in order to maintain an adequate supply of breastmilk.

It may be easier to accept your baby's light sleep if you see this as 'smart sleep', playing an important role in brain development. During active infant sleep, there is an increase in the production of certain nerve proteins – the building blocks of the brain – and blood flow to the brain nearly doubles relative to the deepest sleep state. It is also thought that the brain uses active sleep to process information. This may explain why it is common for babies who have been sleeping well for weeks or months to become wakeful as they enter new developmental stages and practise their new skills such as crawling or standing up. It must be rather like the difficulty we have trying to sleep after a busy day, a big night out or perhaps as we start a brand-new job.

There are a range of factors that can affect your baby or toddler's sleep, including developmental stages: babies tend to wake as they reach significant milestones and these can be physical, emotional or neurological; your child's diet, or your own if you are breastfeeding: food allergy or intolerance, or sensitivity to stimulants such as caffeine or chocolate can cause restlessness which may affect your baby's sleep patterns; dietary deficiencies such as low levels of DHA, an omega-3 fatty acid, are being shown to affect infant sleep patterns, and low iron levels can affect older babies and toddlers' sleep; how much activity is in your child's day (while some babies and children can become easily overstimulated, others benefit from more physical activity and time outdoors to help them sleep more soundly); and your child's sleeping environment can also impact on how well he sleeps.

As you read through this book, you will find a range of options to help you create a positive sleep environment. The responsibility for deciding which options will suit your child and your family is yours. I would urge you though to consider three things as you make your decisions regarding sleep for your baby or child:

- Your child's safety is the number-one prerequisite for making any choices about infant sleeping practices.
- Ask yourself, 'Is this respectful?' and, 'Does it feel right?' We do so many things to small children and babies, without even considering how intrusive or disrespectful it might feel to them. (See Put yourself in their place, page 50.)
- It may be difficult when you are utterly exhausted,

but try to think about the bigger picture and consider what messages you want to send to your child. Will you be teaching your child that sleep is a lovely nurturing space where he is safe to go, and that he can trust you to soothe his fears and mend his hurts whatever the time of day or night? If you can do this, you will not only be investing in sound sleep, but you will be creating a precious bond with your child that will outlast these early sleepless nights.

From the beginning

Good sleep begins at birth. Although a gentle, natural birth experience is no guarantee of a soundly sleeping baby, some interventions can increase the risk of a wakeful baby. You, too, would find it difficult to sleep soundly with a headache or a sore neck or shoulder after a difficult birth experience. The care your baby receives in the early hours and days after birth can help avert feeding problems and subsequent food sensitivities or unnecessary illness due to premature weaning that may cause sleep difficulties weeks or months later. For instance, there is research to show that babies who are taken from their mothers to be weighed and dressed before being allowed to snuggle and breastfeed will be less interested in feeding and may have difficulty suckling.

Immediately after a natural birth, certain hormones that are part of the birth process remain at high levels within your body and your baby's. These play a crucial role in the formation of your relationship: when babies are born free of medication and allowed uninterrupted skin-to-skin contact with their mother (there is no urgency to know your baby's weight or to let Grandma have a cuddle just yet), these hormones will create a high that prepares you and your baby to connect and fall exquisitely in love with each other.

Newborns who snuggle skin to skin (naked against your bare skin) with their mother after birth will usually seek and latch onto the breast without very much help at all, ideally within an hour after birth. If you are patient and allow your baby to take his time, this first breastfeed is usually quite a long suckle lasting anywhere from about half an hour to a couple of hours. Although your baby will only be getting small amounts of colostrum, the early, yellowish fluid which is high in antibodies, this first feed is especially important to help your baby imprint a breastfeeding sucking technique which is different from that required to milk a bottle teat.

Fortunately, whatever your birthing experience, it seems that nature allows more than a single chance to cement the foundation for a loving relationship and to reinforce the bonding process. However you plan to feed your baby or whatever your birth experience, snuggling with your baby against your bare skin as soon as it is practical provides a wonderful start to your relationship: skin-to-skin care will release hormones that help with bonding and attachment as well as boosting your breast-milk. Although bonding with your baby in that 'Wow! I am in love' way can take a few days or even longer to happen, please don't worry – it won't be long and you will be blown away by the deep protective feelings you have for your baby. Honoring your 'mother lioness' instincts to keep your baby close and respond to him will help you develop confidence that you really are the expert on your baby. This confidence will be reflected back to your baby by the way you handle him, giving him a sense of security, and it will stand you in good stead to ignore irrelevant advice, including inappropriate advice about infant sleep.

The first sleeps

After this initial feed, your baby will probably take a long nap. Although there is a wide range of normal, it is quite common for babies to spend the next twenty to twenty-four hours in stages of light and deep sleep. Some babies will wake for short feeds, while others are more sleepy and less interested in feeding.

> Clemmie fed within an hour of birth, but she never did the big long first sleep I was expecting. The longest stretch she did was five hours, otherwise she slept and woke fairly frequently. And she screamed a lot. Perhaps she had a sore head from the ventouse [delivery], or it could have been feeding problems, meaning she was hungry. Who knows, but she still wakes frequently even now. I was expecting lots of sleep from her in the first twenty-four hours, and was fairly shattered myself, so was a bit gutted that she didn't oblige so I could

*get some sleep as well! It was nothing to do with the
hospital – we were at a birth centre for post-natal care,
rooming in, lots of support, consistent advice – I just
had a baby who hadn't read the same books I had.*

Jacqui

*Tiny was one of those good babies (I readily admit this
is the strangest usage of the word 'good' I have ever
encountered) that just slept from day one. When he
was born, I attempted to feed him. He looked at me
for an hour or so then passed out, and spent the first
day sleeping. I was told to wake him up to feed him the
second day.*

*What I tend to see and hear from mums (and this is
what happened with me) is that babies are wide awake
after birth, have a good feed for a long time (say, forty
to ninety minutes), then are sleepy, waking for short
feeds over the next twenty-four hours, then have a feeding frenzy, often sleeping little for the next forty-eight
hours. Another common variation is that the baby is very
passive and will feed when offered, or wake to feed every
three to four hours, but is not proactive about seeking
feeds for the first week. He will be quite hydrated and
feeding well, then wide awake and ratty, sleeping little for
the next week, then into more of a pattern.*

Fiona, midwife

Sleepy babies often cause parents anxiety about whether
to wake their baby for feeds. If you have a hospital birth
there will probably be protocols about how often babies

need to be fed but there is generally no need to worry if your baby takes her time (as long as she has plenty of opportunity through skin-to-skin contact with you). Your baby's stomach will be full of amniotic fluid, and the colostrum she suckled at birth is high in energy and nutrients, so a long sleep at first seems to be nature's way of giving you and your baby time to rest and recover from the enormous task of giving birth.

If you have had medication or complications during the birth, or if you and your baby are separated initially, please be reassured that nature allows ongoing opportunities to bond with your baby and establish feeding, even though this may require extra support. The best thing you can do in the early days is to keep visitors at bay and snuggle with your baby so you can smell, touch and bond with each other. Skin-to-skin cuddles help your baby regulate his body temperature and blood sugar levels and saves him burning unnecessary calories. Skin-to-skin time is especially important if you and your baby are separated at birth, but if you are affected by medication that could reduce awareness of your baby, it is best to have your partner or a support person to supervise and help you handle your baby. With your baby close to you, you will be able to see immediately when he begins to stir and make signals (rooting or sucking movements with his mouth or moving his hand towards his mouth) that indicate he is ready to try feeding.

If your baby isn't interested in feeding or you are separated immediately after birth, you can express some colostrum into a teaspoon and give this to him. If you are reading this before you have your baby, you may like to consider expressing some colostrum in the last few weeks of pregnancy and freezing this in syringes (available at your pharmacy). You can take your frozen colostrum into hospital with you and give this to your newborn if you are advised to give your baby any top-ups because he has low blood sugar, if you are separated after birth, or if your milk takes a little longer to 'come in'.

> I have seen all kinds of sleeping behaviour in unmedicated babies that is normal for the individual babies. In the first day, the baby may feed well about half an hour to an hour after birth and then sleep or not be interested for twelve to twenty-four hours. Subsequently, there may be several days when they are sleepy and not hungry (feeding every five or six hours), then very hungry! Others feed hungrily on and off for the first twenty-four hours and every day thereafter.
>
> Mary, midwife

The first days

After his first day in the world, it is likely that your baby will seem to be making up for lost time as he appears to be wakeful and hungry and even making signs that he is hungry again just a short time after he has been fed. Your baby is likely to be especially cranky on his second night (he's just realised he is 'on the outside'). This wakefulness is not an indicator that you are unable to make enough milk for your baby or that he will have sleeping problems. In fact, this behaviour is so common that it even has a name: cluster feeding.

When this happens, it's very easy to think that a bottle of formula will be helpful. Or you may be offered formula be a well-meaning midwife. However, giving formula now can affect your baby's gut environment and may potentially lead to allergies and ongoing wakefulness. It can also interfere with your body's messages to produce milk. One suggestion to avoid unnecessary formula in these early days is to consider expressing some colostrum during the last few weeks of pregnancy, collecting this in syringes and freezing it. You can take this into hospital with you and give it to your baby if he needs any supplements. It will be a natural boost to your baby's immune system and you will reduce the pressure to give your baby bottles that could create unnecessary breastfeeding challenges. If you are feeling exhausted by your baby's need to feed constantly, it can be helpful for your partner (who won't smell like milk) to snuggle your baby skin to skin to give you a break.

Your newborn has a very tiny stomach and will take very small feeds at first but these early feeds will help your baby learn to breastfeed effectively as he practises coordinating his sucking, swallowing and breathing before he has to deal with large volumes of fluid. Your baby's sucking will also help stimulate your milk production hormones and encourage a healthy milk supply to match his increasing appetite in a few days' time. Then, as he has a nice full tummy, he will take longer sleeps more quickly. There is no sense in trying to impose feeding or sleeping routines during the early days. In fact, by following your baby's cues and feeding frequently, which could be eight to twelve times a day initially, you will be less likely to suffer from uncomfortable breast engorgement, your milk will come in more quickly and milk production will meet your baby's needs.

Jaundiced babies

Jaundice, characterised by a yellowish tinge in baby's skin, is one of the most commonly occurring conditions in babies a few days old. One side effect of jaundice is that babies become very sleepy. However this isn't a time to congratulate yourself for giving birth to a good sleeper, nor is it good practice to let babies with slightly yellow skin sleep for long stretches.

Although some types of jaundice mean your baby will need tests to rule out underlying conditions, the most common jaundice is caused by the baby's immature liver not being able to process and excrete bilirubin, a normal by-product of broken-down red blood cells, quickly enough. The extra bilirubin circulating in your baby's body, causing the yellowish tinge to his skin, is due to the destruction of red blood cells, a normal process after birth.

Since sleepy, jaundiced babies can be difficult to arouse for feeds, leading to more severe jaundice and in turn, more intensive treatment – all the more reason to take preventative measures. Early and frequent breastfeeding without supplements of formula will encourage baby to pass meconium (those first black, tarry bowel motions) and he will more quickly establish good gut flora that will break down bilirubin. So, if your baby isn't waking and demanding to be fed at least by the second day, it is important to wake him and offer feeds at least every two to three hours.

The first six weeks

Just like a honeymoon has traditionally been a time for couples to get to know their partners more intimately, a 'baby moon' is a very special time for you, your partner, if you have one, and your baby – so put aside expectations, shut out the world until you feel ready, and enjoy this precious time getting to know each other and bonding as a family. It is a time to take things slowly and delight in every moment – it takes time and lots of watching to get to know your baby's little quirks and foibles and how he expresses his needs in his own way.

Understanding your baby's needs in these early weeks and creating a healthy sleep environment are the best things you can do to influence your little one's sleep patterns. Although, as the obstetrician Dr Grantly Dick-Read says, your baby has simple needs, all of which can be met in your arms and at your breast, it can help to consider the enormous sensory changes from womb to room from your baby's perspective, and offer 'womb service' as you help your baby adapt to being on the outside.

With newborns, I observe that it takes about a week
for a baby to make the transition from mother's arms
to a bassinette to sleep with any sense of confidence.
A maturation process I am sure.

Karen, midwife

'Womb service' involves re-creating the sensations your baby experienced while he was safely carried inside you. To help you remember the important aspects, I have called these the five Ws:

- Warmth
- Wrapping
- Wearing
- Water
- Womb sounds.

You can use these techniques to help your baby sleep or just to keep her world calm as she makes the transition from womb to room. After all, a calm baby is much more likely to sleep soundly than a stressed baby. To create a healthy sleep environment, you wouldn't necessarily do all of these things at once – for instance, you wouldn't wrap a baby while you are wearing him. Instead, perhaps use one or two things at a time, depending how this works for you and your baby.

Warmth

Inside your body, your baby didn't experience cool air blowing on his tiny body or entering his lungs, and these new sensations can be quite disturbing. So, at first, warm the space where you are going to be with your baby (sixteen to twenty degrees Celsius will be a comfortable room temperature), and take care not to have fans or air-conditioners blowing directly onto him in warmer weather. If you are popping him into a cradle to sleep, he will be more comfortable (and likely to sleep better) lying on sheets that have been warmed slightly. You do need to take care not to overheat your baby, but you can warm his sheets slightly with a heat pack before you place him into bed – test the sheets with your forearm to make sure they aren't hot.

Wrapping

Just as your newborn was tucked snugly inside your body, supported by the uterine wall, you can provide a sense of security by swaddling your newborn – wrapping him in a cotton or muslin sheet (note bunny rugs and blankets can cause overheating) will help your baby feel safe as his limbs are tucked securely (but not tightly) against his body, just as they were in the womb. It may help him stay asleep longer. One reason for this is that a newborn reflex, know as the 'startle reflex', a primitive survival response that produces spontaneous, jerky movements, can be disturbing (literally). Your baby will waken, even from a deep sleep, if his own flailing little arm unexpectedly hits him in the face.

There are several ways to wrap your baby but it's important to consider safety guidelines: Wrap your baby from below the neck to avoid covering his face (see SIDS guidelines on page 108); wrap loosely enough to allow movement and chest expansion and allow room for your baby to move his hips and flex his legs as there are concerns that tight wrapping that restricts movement can contribute to hip dysplasia; dress baby lightly under the wrap to avoid overheating; don't wrap your baby if you are sharing a sleep surface and, as your baby grows, modify the wrap appropriately. For instance, once the startle reflex disappears at around three months, wrap baby with his arms free. And, once your baby can roll over, discard the wrap altogether.

Do unwrap your baby's hands when you feed him so he can touch your skin, or you can hold his tiny hands or kiss his delicate fingers. This will enhance bonding and will also provide extrasensory stimulation as the many nerve endings in his hands and fingers send these powerful 'touch' messages to his brain.

Some mothers find they can 'condition' their babies to differences between day and night by swaddling loosely during the day and wrapping their babies more firmly at night. Be aware that the small wraps most commonly sold will be outgrown very quickly and are often not big enough to securely swaddle even a small baby. It is far better to buy large wraps in the first place.

There are also a number of all-in-one swaddles and swaddle suits on the market. While these can make it much easier to wrap your baby, especially during the night, please take care when buying these that they allow plenty of space for your baby's hip movement. Also consider that when your baby's hand movements are restricted by a tight swaddle, you can't observe his early signals for food such as moving his hand towards his mouth.

As your baby grows, it is better if her movements aren't restricted at all, so a good way to help your little one's transition is to unwrap her body gradually, letting out one arm at a time, then wrapping her with her arms out and later discarding the wrap altogether as the startle reflex disappears around three months. Some babies older than this may sleep better if they are swaddled – follow your baby's lead. If he's more comfortable being swaddled, there is no reason why you can't let him enjoy this security for a while longer. However, it is safer to have your little one unwrapped by about four months so that as he starts rolling, he will not become entangled in his swaddle. It can be a gentle transition to move your baby into a sleeping bag as you discard the wrap. As your baby becomes mobile, a sleeping bag can be a safe way to keep him warm, instead of blankets. Choose a sleeping bag with a fitted neck and armholes that are the correct size for your baby. Also, please read the manufacturer's instructions carefully and choose the correct warmth level on any sleeping bag so you can keep your baby snug without overheating.

Wrapping your baby

Lay the sheet with a corner facing up, to form a diamond shape.

Fold the top corner down towards the centre of the sheet, to form a longer straight edge across the top. Then, if your baby is awake, place him on the sheet with his shoulders near the top, straight edge and draw one side across his body, rolling him a little so you can tuck that edge under his body, leaving his other arm free. Tuck your baby's arms in, one at a time remembering the mantra 'hands to heart'. It's common to be told to wrap your baby's arms down by his side but having his arms up across his chest where he can freely move them (but enclosed by the wrap to inhibit the startle reflex) allows chest expansion, which is important for natural movements that encourage healthy development, as well as for breathing – there is research to suggest that tight wrapping that inhibits expansion of the chest wall can contribute to development of pneumonia.

Fold the bottom point up over your baby's feet and roll the remaining side of the sheet across his body, enclosing your baby's other arm across his chest. As you bring this last point around, you can tuck it into the top of the wrap at your baby's neck or just fold it around behind. Tucking the bottom point up is optional – it depends how long the swaddle is in comparison to your baby.

If your baby has fallen asleep in your arms, gently hold him against your shoulder with one arm and wrap him while you are holding him – lying him flat while he is unwrapped may startle and waken him.

Wearing

On the 'inside', your baby was lulled to sleep by your body movements as you went about your daily work. Now, the motion of being carried in a wrap or front-pack against your moving body and your comforting heartbeat as he breathes your familiar body odours will help your baby feel safe. This feeling of familiarity will reduce stress hormones and help your baby be more relaxed, and a more relaxed baby will sleep more easily. Wearing your baby may have a balancing effect on his irregular rhythms of waking and sleeping and is also thought to help him regulate his developing nervous and hormonal system, promoting day waking and night sleeping.

> Both my children slept on me and in slings during the day for the first three months, and then made the transition to the pram and bassinette gradually, without any stress. They just both screamed if they were separated from me. I can imagine that being inside my womb and then straight into a pram in a prone position was too scary for them. I enjoyed this bonding time, and I could do more things knowing they were safe and comfortable up against me.
>
> Wendy

If your baby falls asleep in the wrap or carrier, you will have two hands free to do a few chores, or you can go out and enjoy a walk. Wearing baby is especially good if you are in a busy, noisy place such as a shopping centre – your motion, as you hold your baby close, will act as a filter for the extra stimulation and help her to sleep through the bedlam. (That said, during the early weeks venues such as shopping centres will probably be stressful to you as well as your baby, so do consider your own wellbeing too.) If you are at home and prefer to put your baby into bed when she has fallen asleep, you can gently slip baby out of most carriers while she is sleeping: simply bend over, lower baby towards the cot and unwrap or unclasp the carrier at the shoulder (depending on the style you have). If you are using a wrap, you can smooth it out under your baby so it isn't a smothering hazard or, depending on the style, wrap it around her safely, rather than try unravelling her completely and risk waking her up.

By using a carrier or wrap in the early days, you will get your body used to your baby's weight before he gets too heavy. It is best to start with short spells at first and gradually carry your baby for longer periods as your muscles adapt.

Safe baby wearing

Just as with any baby equipment, it's important to consider safety precautions when choosing and using a baby carrier. Please make sure you buy from a reputable supplier as there are a number of 'fakes' that have been copied from the better brands, but these can have faulty buckles and unsafe stitching. Also choose a carrier that supports both your baby's and your spine without placing any pressure on your baby's developing hips. Newborns should be carried facing inwards with their legs in a 'froggy leg' position – not 'dangling' down.

Babes in Arms, a reputable Australian sling and carrier

website, says these safety guidelines can be easily remembered by going through the 'Rule of hand'. Each finger represents a different babywearing safety tip, matching the acronym CARRY. By simply learning these five tips, reinforced each time you glance at your hand, you will learn to trust your instincts and enjoy the closeness of your babe.

C-A-R-R-Y

CAREFUL. If you wouldn't do an activity while pregnant, don't do it while wearing your baby. Like being pregnant, babywearing can tilt your centre of gravity and not allow you to see your feet much. Unlike being inside your womb where the baby is protected somewhat, the carried baby does not have inbuilt protection surrounding them. Be mindful of what your baby can reach. Babywearing in the kitchen? Watch the hot pot on the stove or the kitchen knife when you turn to grab something else.

AIRFLOW. You should always be able to easily see your baby's face without opening the fabric. Ensure that your baby's chin is not pressed against her chest to allow easy breathing. To check, simply slip two fingers under baby's chin; when breathing is hindered it could lead to 'positional asphyxia'.

RIDE HIGH. Keep the baby high and tight against your chest, not low on your hips. This will afford you a good line of sight to monitor your baby's needs and wellbeing. You would find it tiring carrying baby in your arms lower than your belly button, likewise a sling that carries your baby low will quickly prove sore on your shoulders and back. A carrier should mimic holding baby in your arms, or in the instance of back carry, like a piggy back.

RIGHT FIT. Make sure that you read your wrap or carrier's instruction booklet and, if available, watch the videos so you can ensure the carrier is the right fit for your body shape and the age and weight of your baby. When trying a new carry position, test it with a doll or teddy the first few times, and with your partner to spot check you. Back carry positions are recommended to learn while kneeling in the middle of your bed.

YOUR INSTINCT. You are the parent, trust your instinct. Try to mimic with the wrap the way you would naturally hold your baby with your arms. You should always be able to make eye contact with your baby. This will allow you to determine whether he is safe, happy and content. A cursory glance will allow you to quickly assess if their chin is up and that they are comfortable.

Water

Help your baby recall his watery womb world by taking a bath together. Remember that on the inside your baby was confined, not floating all stretched out, and his womb world was gently bathed in filtered light. By dimming the lights or bathing by candlelight with your newborn, you will help her recall the safety of her womb world and you will be able to hold her close and support her as she gradually relaxes and uncurls her limbs. Bathing together is especially helpful if bonding has been interrupted by early separation or a difficult birth or feeding experience.

It can also be lovely bonding time for father and baby.

Newborns can lose body heat very quickly after a bath, and a cold baby will be more difficult to settle. So, rather than exposing your baby to cool air by laying her flat on a towel and patting her dry, wrap her in two towels and cuddle her. The heat trapped in the towels will dry most of your baby's body as the warmth relaxes her. Then you can remove the damp towel next to her body and with the outer, dryer towel gently dry her crevices (neck, under-arms, groin, between fingers and toes) and dress her.

To bathe safely with your baby, it is best to have some-body else to help you get in and out of the bath, but if you are on your own, place your baby on a towel that is spread over a baby seat or bouncinette next to the bath. When you are comfortably in the bath, reach over and lift baby in with you. When you need to get out, place baby back in her bouncer, wrap her in the towel to keep her warm while you get dried and pop on your dressing gown, then dress your baby and snuggle together – bliss!

Bathing can be a wonderful sleep cue for babies and children of any age so it can be helpful to introduce an evening bath as one of your earliest sleep associations.

Womb sounds

The calming, repetitive sounds of traditional lullabies recall the 'womb music' your baby heard before birth (your heartbeat, and fluids whooshing through the pla-centa). Baby music that incorporates elements such as the rhythm of a heartbeat or white noise has remarkable soothing effects, especially if played continuously through the night. Of course, your own singing voice or even a gentle, continuous shushing sound is transportable music that doesn't rely on the availability of a device such as an MP3 player and it will help induce calm and sleepiness just as well as any commercial music – even if you don't have a fabulous voice. If you are feeling anxious because your baby is unsettled, you may find it more helpful to hum, rather than sing. Humming will naturally slow your breathing and help you feel calmer. Changing your energy will help soothe your baby since he will be like a little barometer of your own stress levels. Another great tip is to gently bounce on a fit-ball as you hum – your baby will settle more quickly due to the movement and you are toning your bum and thighs as you soothe your little one.

Womb to room

If you have read the information about active and quiet sleep, and how your newborn enters sleep through an active sleep state, you will realise how unrealistic and potentially unsafe it is to expect a tiny baby to self-settle and sleep for long periods, especially if you are expecting her to make this transition without acknowledging the significant sensory changes from the warm softness and perpetual motion of the womb world to a still, flat cot with crisp, cool sheets.

You will now understand how taking a little extra time to assist your young baby into deeper sleep by offering womb service will help her to sleep for a longer stretch. It takes about twenty minutes of active sleep before babies move into a deeper, more restful sleep state, which explains why some babies have difficulty settling or why they may wake again as soon as you put them down if they have fallen asleep in your arms. One tip is to settle your baby in a carrier or in your arms, but wait until his limbs are limp and floppy – a sure sign he has reached a deeper sleep state – before you gently place him in his bed.

Of course, if you prefer to hold him in a wrap or carrier as he sleeps, this is a lovely option too. This is not a time to be concerned about bad habits because, for starters, your baby doesn't have the cognitive skills to manipulate you. Time spent helping your baby adapt to life on the outside is an investment in sound sleep. As your baby feels secure, and as her little nervous system matures through the sensory stimulation of loving touch and movement, she will naturally move from waking to sleep states with less and less assistance; as her stomach capacity increases and she can manage larger quantities of milk at each feed, she will begin to sleep at least one longer stretch in each twenty-four-hour period; and as her trust in you develops it will be easier to help her make changes when you both feel ready.

Mum's the word

You may have planned to carry your baby 'in arms' (in a wrap or front-pack) most of the time, whether he is sleeping or awake. While this closeness is lovely for you and your little one, it can be quite a difficult ideal to live up to in a practical sense. It is common for mothers to feel all touched out from meeting the intense needs of a young baby and it may take a while for your back to feel strong enough to carry your baby for extended periods, so be gentle on yourself and take breaks when you need to. There is a range of options to ease your baby's transition from womb to room without pushing yourself beyond your limits. Remember, you will be more responsive to your baby if you take good care of yourself by balancing your baby's needs with your own.

How does your baby grow?

> *Whenever I held my newborn baby in my arms, I used to think that what I said and did to him could have an influence not only on him but on all whom he met, not only for a day or a month or a year, but for all eternity – a very challenging and exciting thought for a mother.*

Rose Kennedy

Imagining even a few months of broken sleep probably seems like utter torture, especially if you have read all the books that promise you can have a soundly sleeping baby whose nap-times will fit neatly into your organised day. Sadly – or fortunately, depending on how you look at it – much of the stress of trying to force your baby to fit an inappropriate schedule or follow a book that he hasn't read is completely unnecessary. If you work with your baby's natural stages of development, you can save an enormous amount of angst for yourself and your child and you can encourage sleep naturally.

At three months

Between two and three months, your baby will start to see the light of day – literally. Although your baby will need to be fed at least every two to three hours (or sometimes even more often) around the clock in the early weeks, by about eight weeks or so (give or take – this isn't the Baby Olympics!), she will probably now take at least one longer stretch of sleep and, with a little bit of luck and a tiny bit of mummy management, this could be at night. Also, at about eight to twelve weeks, your baby might begin to grasp the difference between day and night and, with a little encouragement, you can work this to your advantage too. (See Feed me, page 154.)

Because your baby will now be more able to stay awake for spells between sleep and feeds, his patterns of sleep and waking will be a bit more predictable. You can help your baby stay awake a little longer between daytime feeds by playing with him, taking him outside (which will help regulate his day–night cycle), keeping him with you as you work and sing and chat to him, although taking care not to let him get overtired. During the day, let your baby sleep in a sling or around the house (take his cradle out into the family room) or wherever the action is, at least for some naps, and keep the curtains open.

At night, a quieter environment will be sleep-inducing: save play and chatter for daylight hours. In the evening, use a dim bedside lamp as you attend to her, keep your movements slow and quiet but please, whatever you do to maintain a dull night-time space, don't avoid eye contact with your baby. I often meet mothers who feel anxious that their babies are not making eye contact and invariably I discover that these mums have been trying to follow a regime where they avoid eye contact with their baby at sleep times or all night, as it has been deemed overstimulating.

But think about it – how do you feel about people who avoid eye contact with you? What if your partner repeatedly avoided your gaze? Eye contact is an important element of bonding and the development of trust between parent and child: your face is the most potent visual stimulus your baby encounters, and as you and your baby gaze into each other's eyes, endorphin levels rise in your baby's brain, producing feelings of joy. Your own endorphin levels will also rise and, in turn, you and your baby become emotionally synchronised. Thankfully, with just a few sessions of deliberate interaction such as infant massage and baby games (and of course, reassurance that mothers haven't inadvertently caused irreparable emotional damage to their child), I have seen mothers and babies reconnect and enjoy their special bond.

When my son Jack (now two) was born I read so many things about rigid routines and how to 'make' babies sleep. Knowing no better I took these things as gospel truth and followed to the letter these routines, despite the fact that they were at times restrictive and upsetting to both of us. I would spend evenings after his 'bedtime' patting, rocking, feeding and attempting to soothe him, without talking to him or making eye contact believing these things would make him more wakeful. We were very lucky in that he was (and still is) an easygoing boy who more often than not would fall asleep quite happily on his own. But on the nights that he couldn't it felt like a personal affront. I couldn't work out why he couldn't just go to sleep like the books said he would if I did these things!

I learned a lot as he got older and realised that I was doing neither of us any justice by taking the word of professed experts over my own basic instincts and intuition.

By the time our daughter, Emma, (five months) was born I had a very different understanding of myself as a parent. I never expected to co-sleep with her having not been successful in doing so with Jack, but from birth she has been a very attached baby and has never spent a night out of my arms.

What an amazing thing! Instead of anxiously waking to cries and getting up to pace while just wishing for sleep, I am able to respond to her movements before she even fully wakes, and feed her back to sleep. On the nights she can't get back to sleep after a feed I am able to talk to and cuddle her, and even look her in the eye! Even in the earliest hours of the morning her smile melts my heart, and it saddens me so much that

I missed out on this amazing and intense night-time relationship with Jack.

Kate

By three months, your baby's attempts at communicating his needs will be much clearer to you, with fewer mixed signals, so hopefully you will find it easier to work with his natural states of alertness and his sleepy signs to make the most of these windows of opportunity to fit fun and sleep into his day (and yours!). Closer to four months, many babies begin to find it easier to fall asleep with very little help, especially if you have begun to create some positive bedtime rituals. (See Time to sleep, page 224.)

Gabby would only fall asleep when on the breast or cuddled. After fighting it for a while, I gave in and decided that if that's what works, then that's the way I was going to do it. It was a relief not to have to stress about what she was meant to be doing. So I just stuck to what worked to get her to sleep. She would only sleep for thirty to forty-five minutes at a time as well. She would sleep out in the bouncer in the lounge room during the day and only sleep in her room at night.

Slowly but surely, Gabby's patterns changed. One day, when she was about four months old, I decided to try to get her to sleep in her room. I put her down once a day in her cradle. She wouldn't sleep for long (and only after I had cuddled her to sleep). One day I had people over and I put her down in her cradle to sleep and she settled herself! I was shocked and rapt at the same time. So I tried it for the next nap and the next. Before I knew it, I had a baby that settled herself and no longer wanted to be fed or cuddled to sleep. All without controlled crying! I had resigned myself to the fact that I would be cuddling her to sleep for a very long time. Now I put her to bed awake.

Debbie Lee

From four to six months

Your baby may now be fairly predictable in his daily pattern, so if you work your day around your baby and include your baby naturally in your daily activities, you are less likely to feel frustrated by interruptions than if you try to impose a rigid schedule that doesn't respect your baby's natural rhythm. Your own energy levels will be returning and although most babies will still need one or two feeds during the night, they feed efficiently and quickly so you will probably manage these feeds with little fuss.

This is why sudden night wakefulness – which can start from around four or five months, even if your baby has been sleeping a good long stretch for weeks – can be quite disconcerting. You worry, what am I doing wrong? When we consider things from a baby's view though, it can make more sense. Babies tend to wake as they enter new stages of development and these can be physical, emotional or neurological.

These changes are often labelled by experts as a 'sleep

regression'. While this explains that something is going on for your baby, this tends to put a negative slant to your baby's normal development. You see, your baby isn't regressing. Sleep isn't a milestone – even though it certainly feels like an achievement when your baby starts snoozing for several hours at a stretch. However, the real, measurable, important milestones that signal your baby's actual development can influence your baby's sleep, or lack of it. So when your baby, who has been sleeping in peaceful blocks, suddenly starts waking more frequently, it usually means he is approaching a real developmental milestone – he is not regressing, he is progressing.

Developmental milestones can be physical (rolling, crawling, cruising, walking), emotional (separation anxiety) and neurological. For instance, at around four months (the four-month sleep regression that everyone is talking about), babies are becoming much more aware of the world. They are babbling, which marks the beginning of language acquisition; they are exploring things with their mouth (soon that will include their feet too as they suck their toes); and many babies are starting to roll over so they wake because they have unintentionally rolled onto their belly. They are confused and upset because they really want to be sleeping but that tiny brain has been processing information, which has resulted in some extra practice of their new skill. All of this adds up to a very busy little brain that finds it difficult to switch off. And, as well as often having difficulty getting to sleep in the first place or resettling after being woken by their busy brains and bodies, when he wakes, confused, your baby will call for help from the most important person in his world – you.

Neurological milestones are outlined in *The Wonder Weeks*, a book by Dutch researchers, psychologists Frans Plooij and Hetty van der Rijt, who observed many children in their homes over a number of years. They describe the wonder weeks as critical periods of development that change the baby's perception of his world. For instance, at twenty-six weeks babies start to perceive distance. This means that as you walk away, your baby is now more aware of the distance that separates you, and he will yell at you because the increasing distance between you and him is confusing and a bit scary.

Around this time, too, a new emotional milestone of separation anxiety is beginning. For some babies this starts earlier but whenever it happens it is an exciting indication that your baby is very well connected to you – you are his rock and the most important person in his whole world, so this is why he is likely to get upset as you move out of sight or pass him to somebody else to hold. At this stage, he hasn't developed what psychologists call 'object permanence', which means that he doesn't yet understand that when you disappear you will come back again – or that you even still exist. Understandably, this can be quite unsettling for some babies and explains why they often start to become clingy and wake, possibly for reassurance. Some parents find it helpful at this stage to 'leave a bit of mum' as baby sleeps: slip your own soft, unwashed t-shirt over baby's mattress. Although it's not exactly a substitute for you, she will be comforted by your familiar smell as she sleeps.

Although a baby of any age can be a bit hungry as he goes through a growth spurt and therefore need extra feeds for a few days, or a six-month-old baby may seem insatiable as he becomes ready to eat solid foods, there are other factors to consider. (See Feed me, page 154.) This is a very exciting stage for your baby with lots of new experiences due to his increasing mobility and awareness, and days can be so stimulating that night may be the only time he can really concentrate on feeding quietly, so it is very common for babies this age to need longer or more frequent feeds at night.

Of course if your baby suddenly becomes unsettled or wakeful at any time, it's important to check that there isn't a medical reason or an impending illness such as sore ears or a urinary tract infection (babies generally wake when they wee if they have a UTI because it hurts). If your baby has recently started family foods, it's also worth ensuring she isn't upset by food sensitivities.

Once you have ruled out illness as a reason for sudden changes in your baby's sleep patterns, consider your baby's development: what new skills is your baby learning? Is she a bit more clingy during her awake times? Does she seem more sensitive right now? And try to see her wakefulness as a positive – she is not regressing, she is progressing. She is learning and developing in leaps and bounds. She isn't waking because you have done anything wrong. You aren't encouraging bad habits, you are helping your baby feel secure as she grows through these intense developmental stages. You don't have to justify your baby's behaviour with fancy labels or reasons for her waking (except to yourself, perhaps, if it makes you feel better).

The good news is that as your baby masters each new milestone there will be spells of sound sleep again – until the next developmental leap!

From six to twelve months

This new stage of needing mummy nearby won't go away overnight. It will, in fact, get even stronger over the next few months, peaking between nine and twelve months and tapering towards about eighteen months, although some children are anxious about separation for up to three years.

All you can really do to help your little 'velcro baby' is to reassure her with your presence. As you move out of sight, talk to her so she can hear you are still near and create 'goodbye' and 'hello' rituals if you do need to leave her with a babysitter so she gradually learns that you will always come back. At sleep times this may translate to staying with your baby until she falls asleep or sleeping with her next to you, either in your bed for part of the night or in her cot next to your bed where you can easily reach out and reassure her.

As your baby develops new skills such as crawling and pulling herself up on her feet she will probably practise these newfound skills in her sleep. This processing of new information is apparently fabulous for infant brain development, even if it means parents will be woken by babies bumping into the sides of cots several times a night. You will need to check on your baby and settle her again. If she has pulled herself up on the side of the cot, she isn't being naughty by refusing to lie down again. Chances are, an inbuilt baby reflex (the symmetrical tonic neck reflex) is preventing her from getting down again. Until this reflex goes, when your baby's legs are straight her head will be bent forward (looking at you over the bars of her cot!), then as she puts her head back (perhaps as you come into her room) her knees will bend and she will sit down again – thump!

One tip that parents of mobile babies find helpful is to settle baby on a large mattress on the floor, rather than in the cot. You can leave her to sleep on the mattress as long as the room is childproofed and, with more room to wriggle around, she may sleep longer without disturbing herself – or you!

Your baby will probably be getting teeth and will have started eating solid foods, and when we add all of these experiences together – practising new skills, a bit of discomfort from teething, and unfamiliar tummy sensations from eating food – you can see why some babies may need help with settling and sleeping again, even if they have been relatively 'good' in the past few months.

Try not to make developmental comparisons with other babies. Each baby will develop nicely at his own speed and you will find that while one baby is concentrating on a physical skill such as crawling or walking, another may be saying a few words or doing tricks such as clapping hands, waving or blowing kisses. Eventually all babies will master these skills, whichever order it happens.

From twelve to eighteen months

I find a lot of parents become quite disheartened about their baby's waking at this age. They feel they have followed the baby's lead for a whole year (or more!) and there seems no sign that this child will ever sleep all night. Often this brings dissent between partners as one exerts pressure to 'make that child sleep' and the other loses faith that the toddler will ever sleep without desperate measures – namely, controlled crying.

In fact, this is a disastrous age to leave babies to cry it out, as separation anxiety is at a peak at about twelve months, and after all the work you have done teaching your baby to trust you, the light is just around the corner (honestly!), even if you do nothing at all but continue to respond to your baby with love. If you are exhausted and fractious, you will feel better to know you can make changes sensitively without leaving your baby to scream, so it is best to work together with your partner if you have one and make a plan of action if changes are in order. (See Sleep: one step at a time, page 248.)

Taliver is fourteen months and the clinginess is starting to drive me bananas! Even when I try to give him to his

*dad, his fists clench and he suctions himself to my body
and I have to try to peel him off me. He's fine once he's
with another person, unless he can see me. When we
are visiting my mum or someone else, he can be playing
perfectly happily by himself or with one of my younger
sisters, but if I walk in the room he bursts into tears and
has to be held (by me and only me of course!).*

*At least he usually likes to sleep alone so I get a bit
of time to be me (and only me). I do enjoy it when he
nestles into me, but those moments are few and far
between. I think he gets frustrated because he is torn
between wanting to be with me, and wanting to explore
everything.*

Michelle

The only constant in the young toddler's day is change.
As he moves through the developmental stages from
crawling to walking to running, his world is expanding at
an incredible rate. He may also be experiencing separations such as childcare for the first time, so it is perfectly
natural for him to want to keep you in his sights as he
ventures forth into the exciting world beyond your lap.
Be patient with your clingy toddler – the quickest way
to help him become independent is to meet his needs for
security. You can encourage independence but pushing
him beyond his limits will usually result in more clingy
behaviour.

If you do need to leave your toddler, don't ever try
to sneak away. Be honest and create goodbye and hello
rituals so that she learns that although you may leave her

for short periods, you will return. At first, practise this ritual as you leave the room and let her play by herself for short periods. It may also help to try short separations by waving goodbye as your child goes out with another familiar person such as grandma for a short walk – often toddlers are happy to leave you, rather than be left.

You may need to sit in your toddler's room, perhaps with a hand on him, as he falls asleep – don't try to force him to self-settle before he is ready, as bedtime should never be associated with stress.

Your toddler's separation anxiety could mean that for a while he may want only one parent to put him to bed. It's most common for babies to initially prefer mum – after all, she is usually the one who feeds and nurtures more of the time so is more likely associated with comfort and familiarity. Also, until around two, babies see themselves as an extension of mum.

Toddlers can show a preference for either parent. You might have been giving and giving to your child all day but as soon as the other parent walks in the door, it's squeals and laughter and you feel like a rotten old piece of meat. Parent preference is a normal stage of development for babies, toddlers and preschoolers and it isn't just about exerting control. At this stage, the frontal cortex is not yet fully developed and they can only manage to focus on one relationship at a time. Often too, a parent preference can be due to routines that we have implemented for convenience, such as who puts the children to bed. If your baby has been breastfed to sleep or your toddler is usually in bed before your partner gets home, you can gently help your little one to accept changes by including your partner in parts of the bedtime routine, such as bathing or massage or helping with naps during weekends, and gradually increasing their involvement. As your baby's separation anxiety eases, the other parent can try settling him.

We can't force children's development by pushing them onto the other parent or punishing them for our own hurt feelings. In fact, this can backfire as they start seeing you as the grumpy parent and your partner as the nice one. We also need to respect littlies' capacity to manage relationships and switch from one parent to another. For instance, if your child wakes in the night and needs comfort from one parent, this isn't the time to insist the other parent will fix it. This is about your child's security and sense of trust that his comfort person is there for him when he is scared or hurt.

If your child has a parent preference right now, you and your partner can work together to encourage strong relationships with both parents. Take heart, as children grow, they will work out ways to connect with both parents all by themselves.

If their toddler is experiencing separation anxiety, some parents find that giving their toddler a transitional object such as a soft toy can be a comfort, too. If you do this, try to avoid using the comfort object as a substitute for your attention. Plan to have two or three of the same objects in case one gets misplaced and alternate these so they all have the same smell, otherwise the new object may be rejected.

About now, many babies will start to drop a daytime sleep, so that soon they will be having just one sleep during the day. The transition between dropping sleeps can be a tricky balance of managing sleep times so that your baby is ready for bed at a reasonable time: sometimes she will need an extra sleep late in the afternoon (or she may fall asleep in the car, for instance) and this may make bedtime later some nights. If your child is still having two daytime naps at this stage and this means her bedtime is quite late, you may be able to tweak her day sleeps so she drops down to one. Gradually move her morning nap later, until it becomes one midday nap.

Typically, toddlers are ready to wake as soon as the first ray of sunshine hits the window and this can be more pronounced as they reach new developmental milestones such as starting to walk. Black-out blinds or dark coloured curtains may help extend your toddler's morning wake-up time, and a sippy cup of water and a few safe toys or board books within reach next from the bed or cot may buy you a few extra minutes if your child will amuse himself for a while when he wakes. If it seems that early morning noise from the street could be waking your toddler, you could set a clock radio either on a station that plays classical music or between stations so it plays white noise. If it starts to play before your child would normally wake, this might help him sleep through the early-morning street sounds. But please remember to keep the volume low to avoid any potential damage to hearing.

> An issue that my mother's group talks a lot about is
> their toddlers waking early. I say to them that I feel
> there is nothing more special than having my little boy
> run in to our bed and come in for another cuddle. He
> knows he is always welcome in our bed. They look at me
> strangely. I know the other mothers have been locking
> their door, their toddler's door, walking them back to
> their bed, leaving toys in their room; anything to get
> more sleep. I say, why not one more relaxed cuddle in
> the morning, rather than beginning the day upset for
> both parent and child.
>
> Molly

From eighteen months

As your toddler becomes more mobile, life is often far too exciting to interrupt by going to bed – at least that seems to be the lively child's perspective! This is when a predictable rhythm to the day and a gentle wind-down ritual before bed becomes vital to help your child switch off from her busy day.

Try to finish boisterous games early in the evening, turn off the television and create a calm, quiet time before bed. An increased understanding and emerging language skills will make bedtime rituals gradually easier as story-time becomes a welcome part of the evening.

Many parents tell me that after close, hands-on bedtime parenting, they feel confident that little ones between eighteen months and two years are ready for some limit-setting around bedtimes and, possibly because the child's needs have been so well met, changes seem to be made fairly easily without any distress to the child or guilt and angst for the parents. However, it's important to bear in mind that night-waking will still be common during the second year and even longer: toddlers still have lots of REM sleep so dreams and possibly even nightmares can influence sleep (and night-waking); some children are bothered by teething – think molars – and if you are having another baby now, you can expect disturbances to your toddler's sleep as he adjusts to changing family dynamics. Whatever the reasons for night-waking at this age, by offering comfort you will move through challenges far more quickly than if you create bedtime battles, as your little one will feel secure.

Two to three years

Delaying bedtime becomes an art at this stage. These little people like to be where the action is and they seem to have no idea they aren't miniature adults. The good news is that your very active, wriggly toddler will enjoy snuggling and listening to a bedtime story and, generally closer to three years, a meditation is a sure way to help him drift off relaxed and with pleasant dreams. (See Time to sleep, page 224.)

Your toddler's delaying tactics – needing a drink, one more kiss, a lost toy – are her way of saying, 'I really want you to stay with me.' From a toddler's perspective, it may be difficult to relax and fall asleep if she feels stressed about being left in her room alone, especially if she can hear adults having fun (talking, watching television) in another part of the house. Consider also if this is the only time of her – and your – busy day that your little one has your undivided attention. If this is the case, try to spend more one-on-one time with her during the day so her needs aren't so intense at bedtime.

A consistent bedtime routine with specific rituals is important to enlist your toddler's cooperation and help him feel secure. Tell him how many stories you will read before you start and to minimise delaying tactics and calling out, try to anticipate his needs. For instance, before he gets into bed, let him get his toys in order and perhaps choose a soft toy to sleep with, place a lidded cup of water within his reach (juice is not good for tiny teeth) and, before you settle down to read, ask him, 'What is the one last thing you need to do before stories?' Help your child stay in bed until he is sleepy by sitting in his room with him. One lovely ritual is to lead him through a relaxation exercise by quietly saying goodnight to each of his body parts and telling him to feel them becoming heavy and sleepy. Start at the toes, move to the legs, knees, tummy and so on, up to, 'Goodnight, sleepy eyes.' If he talks, remind him in a quiet, calm voice that it is sleep time.

There are also some lovely relaxation audio stories for children – have a look at Dinosnores (dinosnores.com.au). Your child will still need cuddles and connection time with you but the audio stories can help you gently wean off staying with your toddler until he falls asleep. If you have things you need to do or you are moving to the next stage of helping your child get to sleep by himself (he will probably need to be close to three years before this will work), you could tell him, 'I just need to go to the toilet/get into my pyjamas/feed the dog, then I will come straight back.' It is important to keep this promise so that he relaxes, knowing you will be back soon. Then, stay with your little one until he falls asleep. Over a few nights you can gradually increase the time you are out of his room and soon he will be falling asleep before you get back and you will be able to tell him, 'I will pop back and check on you when you are asleep.'

At this age, one possible reason for night-waking can be 'bladder awareness' – in other words your little one may be waking to wee. If your child is now going to the potty during the day, a simple thing to do is a 'dream wee'. Just before you go to bed, lift your sleepy tot and carry him to the toilet. Sit him there and in a quiet voice say, 'Do a wee.' Keep the lights dim, snuggle your child and tuck him back into bed. With luck, he will arouse without waking fully, wee in the toilet and go back to sleep – until a reasonable hour.

As imagination is coming on board, your child may wake from a scary dream. Respect your little one's fears – they are real to her. Hold her and reassure her, 'I am here, you are safe.' Stay as long as she needs you and if she is wide awake, or perhaps during the day when she is more likely to be rational, you could tell her, 'When I was little I used to have scary dreams too but I learned to change the end of dreams so they aren't scary anymore.'

Help her think of ways to beat the scary creatures she dreams about. For instance, creating a special sound that makes snakes disappear or using a spray that evaporates monsters or makes them into friendly monsters. A night-light or a dream-catcher (to catch scary dreams) hung above your child's bed may help her feel more confident about going to sleep if she has experienced nightmares, and do consider the role television can play in creating frightening images to a small child.

> Since Jeremy was very little, Cameron and I would sit in two recliner chairs, read books, say prayers and let Jeremy lay with us until he fell asleep, while Cameron and I chatted about our day. Before Samuel was born, Jeremy would always fall asleep with us talking, which I imagine was very soothing for him. Since Samuel has been born, he has joined the tradition happily and we are each able to give our boys a long, relaxed, end-of-the-day cuddle . . . These days, after a little while, Jeremy will either ask to go to bed or we will say it is time for bed and he will happily let us put him in bed awake and he will fall asleep. Bedtime is a happy, calm and peaceful time for all of us. I also believe that with Jeremy being two and very busy playing through the day, we know that we will at least get in a warm snuggle each night which is very special and so important.
>
> **Larissa**

In their own time

As you can see, there is a wide variation in what is normal development for babies and toddlers, and this is reflected by the variation in sleep patterns. There is no point becoming frustrated as the baby next door sleeps all night before yours. At times, it may seem as though the only baby who 'sleeps like a baby' is somebody else's child. But take heart, chances are when your baby 'gets it', your neighbour's child may have a few bad nights. Infant development means lots of changes and ups and downs, but with patience and a few sensible strategies, you will be able to create a healthy sleep environment that respects your baby's developmental needs as well.

Where does your baby sleep?

'Western cultures are unique in the amount of physical separateness which they impose on infants, inventing innumerable gadgets – prams, cots, baby chairs and bouncers.'

Penelope Leach, psychologist

In many cultures parents would never be faced with the question, 'Where will our baby sleep?' These babies would sleep snuggled against the warm body of their mother. However, a quick peep in any baby magazine or local baby store is enough to create confusion for the most assured parent in our modern society – bassinette (how long will my baby fit in one?), cot (practical, pretty or both?), hammock (but how do we change to a cot later?). Can my baby sleep in a pram, a capsule or a stroller? Is it okay to look a gift horse in the mouth when it comes to second-hand baby bedding? Or should we accept all offers? Could we bypass equipment altogether and make up a family bed?

When I was a young single woman and working as a nurse (not yet a midwife) I was fortunate enough to work in the Northern Territory for a couple of years. (Later, after marrying, I went back and worked there for another six years.) I ended up in Nhulunbuy on the Gove Peninsula in East Arnhem Land at a tiny hospital there, which mainly catered to the Aboriginal population.

I spent a lot of time working with the paediatric patients who were generally little bubs with chest infections. We always had mother boarders with children. The Aboriginal mothers and babies always slept together. Usually the baby was brought down on to the mattress on the floor with the mother. They were all breastfed if they were under two or often older.

As a nurse I was amazed at how easy this made my job! The babies were happier (you know how unhappy sick babies can be) and usually didn't cry at all. I also started to see that these mums carried their babies all day or sat with them but didn't leave them for long, breastfed them frequently (sometimes constantly) and were very caring and loving towards their children. I started to think that these mums seemed to be on to a good thing as you hardly ever heard the babies cry and they all seemed so happy and in love with each other. I later spent several years as a midwife in the area and learned so much about breastfeeding from these women.

So before I ever even got pregnant I had decided that our babies (we've had three) would not sleep alone and that co-sleeping seemed much more natural and convenient. Luckily my husband is a very cooperative type and was happy to go along with my ideas. We have always had a futon and, after having our children, had to upgrade it to a king size to keep it comfortable. I also bought a baby hammock and used it intermittently in the first few months, and also a little rocker chair thing – I preferred that as you could move it around the house or outside when you were doing things while they were asleep.

Maxine

From birth, each of our babies slept in a bassinette in our bedroom. I found this the easiest arrangement for us as I could hear when they woke up and could take them into bed to feed and then settle them. When I had Harry (our first) I was paranoid about having him sleep in the bed with us and I ended up spending a lot of time rocking and soothing him at night, as in his first weeks he was a generally unsettled newborn and also colicky.

When we brought Grace home I had no such qualms about her sleeping in bed with us. Being our second baby I was a lot more relaxed with her and she was relaxed too I think. I would put her down to sleep in the *bassinette and when she woke at night I would feed her in our bed, then if she went back to sleep I would put her back in the bassinette. If she was looking like she wanted to stay awake I would settle her next to me in bed in the crook of my arm and we would both go comfortably off to sleep. She grew too big for the bassinette at around four months so I moved her into the cot in her own room. She has been fine in there and settles well at night. We also did this with Harry. Our bedroom is not big enough to fit the cot and we felt that it was better for them to have their own space for sleeping.*

This has worked well for us, although around the time Grace was born Harry started refusing to sleep in his room and screamed if we left him so he started sleeping on the floor in our bedroom at night. He did this up until a week ago when we finally transferred him back to his little bed in his bedroom, and he has handled that well and now goes off to sleep on his own. He is older now, though, and he has had time to adapt to Grace being around and I think he is finally feeling secure again.

Bonnie

The best place for any baby to sleep is where she sleeps best and will depend on your individual family situation.

Having said this, I would like to qualify that the first consideration for any sleeping baby is her safety. Wherever your baby sleeps, it is important to maintain a safe sleeping environment. It is especially important to bear in mind that when we are exhausted it is easy to lose perspective and do whatever works without taking the time to do safety checks, and this is when accidents can happen. For instance, leaving a baby asleep on a sofa, or sleeping with your baby on a sofa is not a safe sleeping environment as babies can fall onto the floor, become wedged in crevices or wriggle under cushions which may impede the baby's breathing.

Reducing the risk of SIDS or SUDI

One of the greatest fears for parents is the possibility of SIDS, sudden infant death syndrome, also known as cot death, or SUDI, the sudden unexplained death of an infant. SUDI may be the result of a serious illness or a problem that baby may have been born with, but most SUDI deaths occur as a result of either SIDS or a fatal sleep accident. SIDS is defined as the sudden, unexpected death of a baby or child for no apparent reason. There is no single cause of SIDS, but experts have identified risk factors and recommend safe sleeping practices that have dramatically reduced its incidence. SIDS and Kids 'Safe Sleeping' is an evidence-based health promotion campaign developed in conjunction with local and international researchers that provides information about SIDS risk reduction and fatal sleeping accidents.

Check with the SIDS or SUDI organisation in your country for the latest safety guidelines as new research is published and updated.

Whatever the triggering mechanisms for SIDS, these can be minimised by breastfeeding your baby as well as safe sleep practices. These include sleeping your baby on his back with his head and face uncovered and maintaining the safest possible environment: avoid exposure to cigarette smoke before and after birth; sleep within proximity of your baby – in the same room as you for the first six to twelve months; do not put your baby to sleep on a soft surface, such as a couch, beanbag or waterbed; never leave your baby unattended in an adult bed or asleep in a pram. Use a cot that meets the current Australian standard.

Back to sleep

The safest sleeping position for babies is on their backs. If a baby's face is nuzzled into bedding, this can hinder breathing: babies wake naturally if their oxygen level decreases, but it is unclear whether the SIDS risk factor is the challenge to the baby's breathing or the baby's response to this.

Lying face down with his face pressed into the mattress may also increase your baby's contact with bugs that thrive in the warm, moist environment of the bed. Research carried out by Dr Richard Jenkins, a senior lecturer in microbiology at De Montfort University in the UK, has identified a link between SIDS and bacteria that breeds in babies' mattresses. He suggests that bacteria may be implicated in up to 50 per cent of SIDS cases. The bacteria seem to thrive on moisture (from vomit or urine) in water-soluble material in polyurethane foam filling, and concentrations were a hundred-fold higher if the baby had been fed formula rather than breastmilk.

The research confirmed that the abundance of bacteria rose with the number of babies that had used the mattress, which may explain why SIDS is more common among second and subsequent babies who may be using a hand-me-down mattress.

SIDS and Kids advise to use a firm, clean mattress that is the correct size for the cot. The mattress should not be tilted but rather should sit flat. Best practice is for a firm mattress. In 2013 an Australia/New Zealand standard was published, the first such sleep surface firmness advice in the world. For your own peace of mind, before you purchase a mattress or product to sleep baby on, you can ask, 'Is this product compliant with the Voluntary Standard AS/NZS 8811.1:2013?'

Use a washable mattress cover. Wash the mattress with soap and water, not chemical cleaners, check for nicks in the covering that could allow moisture to enter the mattress filling, and air your baby's mattress regularly (the same goes for pram mattresses).

If your doctor advises you to put your baby to sleep on his tummy or side to alleviate a particular medical condition, they will explain what precautions to take. If you are advised to put your baby to sleep on his side, keep the lower arm well forward to stop him rolling onto his tummy, or perhaps you could use a baby sleep wrap such as Safe T Sleep, which is specifically designed to maintain a safe sleeping position. When your baby is awake, encourage tummy time to strengthen neck and shoulder muscles. Even newborns can be placed on their tummies for short periods – at first, lying on your chest as you lean back. Later, you can lay baby across your lap and stroke her back, or place her on the floor with a rolled towel beneath her chest for support (with her arms forward) and lie down and talk to her or show her toys. Later she will love watching her reflection in a mirror as she lies on her tummy. Strong head and neck control may help babies lift their heads and roll away if they are finding breathing difficult.

An uncovered head

Overheating poses a risk to babies and as excess heat is lost through the scalp, don't put a hat on your baby for sleep. It is also vital to keep your baby's face uncovered during sleep. Use natural fibre bedding that can breathe, and tuck bed coverings in securely so baby can't slide under them. In a cot, prevent your baby from sliding down under bedclothes by placing him 'feet to foot' – with his feet at the bottom end of the cot – and just make up this half of the bed.

No pillows or soft toys

Do not use quilts, doonas, pillows or cot bumpers for babies under a year old, and do not place soft toys where baby sleeps. Please don't use those soft toy comforters that have a head and a fabric skirt. Apart from the fact that your baby needs *you* at this age, not an inanimate comfort object, these can become a suffocation hazard. (I have seen toddlers with protruding teeth from having sucked on knots on the corners of their beloved comforter.) If your older baby has a snuffly nose and a health professional suggests slight elevation to make breathing easier, place a folded towel *under* the mattress or prop the head of the cot up on phone books.

No butts

Keep your baby smoke-free before and after birth: the risk of SIDS is increased if the mother smokes during pregnancy or after the birth. It isn't simply the inhalation of cigarette smoke by the baby that is an issue. New evidence suggests that the development of a baby's arousal mechanism in his brain is affected by exposure to tobacco smoke during pregnancy. This means that even if you don't smoke near your baby after he is born, if you smoke during pregnancy you have already predisposed your baby to risks that he may be less likely to arouse if he does encounter a breathing problem. There is also evidence to suggest that a father smoking during his partner's pregnancy increases the risk of SIDS, and if both parents smoke the risk is doubled. In fact, do not let anyone smoke near your baby, especially inside the house or in a car.

If you want to quit smoking and you're not finding it easy, ask for help. Call Quitline or ask your doctor, midwife or child health nurse for information and advice.

Sharing a room

A comprehensive New Zealand study on SIDS showed one-fifth the risk of death for sleeping infants sharing the same room with non-smoking adults, and in the largest ever study of cot death it was found that over half the deaths (52 per cent) might have been prevented if the baby had slept in the parents' room.

This protective effect does not work if the baby is in the room with other children, probably because the children wouldn't know if the baby is safe or not. However, parents, especially a mother who is hormonally programmed to be aware of her baby, can check on a baby who is close to her and will be aware of nuances in her baby's noises and movement. She will easily arouse to attend to her baby if he needs help. Recent evidence from the UK indicates that sharing the same room during baby's daytime sleeps is also protective. This doesn't mean you need to shut yourself in the bedroom every time your baby naps but it does explain why many mums feel more comfortable having their young baby sleep in a room where they are, such as the kitchen or lounge room, during the day.

Medication

A wakeful baby is safer than a medicated baby. It is inappropriate to give babies a nightly dose of infant Panadol or similar over-the-counter medications in an attempt to induce sleep. Excessive or prolonged dosage of such medications may be harmful to your baby's immature liver and kidneys and sedating your baby will deprive her of active sleep, which she needs for growth, memory and learning.

If baby's waking is due to a medical condition such as reflux, which may be helped by appropriate medication, or if you suspect your baby may be unwell, please check with your health care provider.

Sleeping in different positions

Although placing your baby to sleep on his back reduces the risk of SIDS, it is necessary to change your baby's position to avoid the development of positional plagiocephaly, the medical name for a misshapen or asymmetrical head shape or, to be perfectly blunt, a flattened head.

Often newborns have funny-shaped heads due to their position in the womb or perhaps some moulding as they were being born, but by about six weeks after birth your baby's head will have regained a lovely round shape. However, because the bones in his head are thin and flexible, if your baby lies with his head in the same position for too long his head can develop a flat spot.

To avoid a flattened head, when you put your baby to bed on his back, gently turn his head to alternate sides each time he sleeps. Moving his cot around so your baby turns his head to look in different directions at his surroundings will encourage him to change positions too. And when your baby is awake, rather than leaving him to play on the floor while lying on his back under a mobile for long periods, or keeping him restricted in an infant seat or car seat that will press against his tiny head, it is very important to encourage tummy time. Tummy time when your baby is awake will help your baby develop a strong upper body and shoulder muscles that will prepare him for rolling (especially if he encounters any breathing obstructions during sleep) and crawling, then later for being upright ready to walk.

You can start giving newborns time on their tummies by laying your baby against your chest as you lie back and relax. In a few weeks your baby will enjoy a gentle back massage as he lies across one of your legs on his tummy or, as he gets better at holding his head up, you can lie on the floor opposite your baby and talk to him – at first, support his chest with a rolled-up towel placed under his arms (place his arms forward across the towel). Later, your baby will enjoy looking at himself in a mirror or playing with toys as he lies on his tummy.

And so to bed

Your baby's bed can be as elaborate as an heirloom cradle (so long as it meets current safety standards) or as simple as a small patch of space alongside you in your own bed.

Hammocks

There is a range of options for baby beds and it can be quite confusing, but if you consider your baby's perspective it may help as you explore your options. In the earliest days, your baby will probably sleep more soundly in an environment that makes the womb-to-room transition easier, so you may like to take a look at baby hammocks and cradles which are suspended so that as the baby moves, he starts his bed rocking or swaying, much like how he was lulled to sleep while he was in the womb. Just like a traditional bassinette, the modern versions of these rocking cradles have a flat mattress so baby can be safely placed on his back to sleep, and while some can be suspended from a hook in the ceiling, others have stands so that you can easily move your baby around the house. Bear in mind that there isn't an Australian safety standard for hammocks so, to ensure your baby's safety, check whether the hammock you are considering has a safety approval certification from another country. Also, do your homework regarding any reports of accidents associated with particular hammocks and check carefully that there are no tipping or falling risks, especially as your baby becomes mobile.

We used hammocks (hanging from the roof) for our twins. We thought having two babies to settle when crying or unwell might just be easier with hammocks, which turned out to be right. They're also a great space saver. Our girls absolutely loved their hammocks. They were in them until they were almost twelve months old. We would happily have kept them in hammocks except they were rolling over and getting stuck wanting to sleep on their tummies so we thought it best to move into cots.

Our girls – Amy and Sarah – settled themselves back to sleep when they awakened (as they often do when so young) with the gentle rocking motion from the hammock. Hammocks are also fantastic for colic or unwell babies. Our girls suffered from wind which was sometimes quite severe resulting in a three-hour process to relieve the pain. They also had silent reflux

*and various allergies. We found the hammocks helped a
lot with settling them.*

Melinda

Cradles and cots

If you are offered a loan of an older-style rocking cradle
or this happens to be your family heirloom, please do a
safety check, especially noting spaces between bars – are
these compliant with current standards, so your baby isn't
at risk of getting her head or limbs stuck? Also, whether
the cradle can be locked into place so it won't rock unless
you are present – babies have been known to rock themselves into a corner and become stuck in unsafe positions.

You may decide that your baby will grow so quickly
that it isn't worth buying a cradle. This is a perfectly reasonable option, but if you put your baby straight into a cot,
remember the SIDS guidelines of putting your baby feet
to foot and only making up the end of the bed where your
baby sleeps. While she is little, your baby could sleep in a
'moses basket' placed in the cot or you could use a sleeping
bag instead of blankets so your baby keeps snug and warm
without the possibility of sliding under the blankets.

Modern cots are height adjustable, so you can have the
base of the cot positioned so your baby is at a higher level
in the cot when he is tiny, then lower the base down as your
baby grows and becomes mobile. As soon as your baby can
climb out of his cot – or it looks like a possibility – he is
ready to be moved to a big bed.

One way to make sure the cot you are buying complies
with strict safety guidelines is to look for the Australian

Standard logo. This will usually be included on the product label but if you aren't sure, ask the retailer. It is illegal in Australia to sell or hire either new or second-hand household cots that don't meet the Australian Standard. Other countries will have their own standards regulations and regulatory bodies.

A co-sleeper cot

There are several brands of cots that can be attached to your bed so that you can sleep in proximity to your baby while the baby also has her own safe sleep space. Many parents find this makes night feeds very easy – you don't even have to get out of bed and you can respond to your baby as soon as she signals, meaning you can feed and settle your baby very quickly. So far there are no Australian Standards for co-sleeper cots. The world's only safety standard specifically written for bedside sleepers is the ASTM Bedside Sleeper Standard. While you may decide to save money by pushing any cot against your bed, it's important to check that the cot can't move away from the bed, creating gaps that your baby can be trapped in and that the cot is at a level that prohibits your baby from rolling into your bed without you being aware. At least in the early months, it is probably safer to use a specially designed co-sleeper bed that meets safety standards, attaches securely and is height adjustable to your own bed.

Safety at home

- Do not place the cot near windows, heaters or power points. This will reduce the risk of injuries from strangulation (from curtains or cords), falls, burns and electrocution.
- Check the cot regularly for signs of wear. Repair peeling paint or transfers immediately as a child may swallow and choke on these.
- Remove climbing aids such as large toys, cot bumpers and cushions from the cot once the child can stand.
- Do not allow small objects to be placed in the cot or anywhere within reach of the child. These could cause the child to choke.
- Make sure the space above the cot is free of objects such as pictures or mirrors that could fall on the child.
- Make sure bases on adjustable base cots are moved to their lowest setting as soon as the child is able to sit unaided.
- Do not place mobiles or toys with cords in cots.
- Do not place soft, fluffy products such as pillows, comforters or sheepskins under infants while they sleep.
- Do not use V- or U-shaped pillows for children under two years of age. Small children can become wedged in the pillow and suffocate. It is safer not to use a pillow at all for children under two.
- Never use electric blankets or hot-water bottles for babies or young children.

Portable cots

Portable cots need to be correctly assembled to prevent them collapsing. Check for dual locking mechanisms to prevent accidental release of locks and collapse of the cot sides onto your sleeping baby. Always use the mattress attached to the portacot and never add additional mattresses or cushioning: this can create gaps between the added mattress and the flexible sides of the portacot that can become a suffocation hazard. The safety standards for portacots published in 2010 introduced new requirements for a breathability zone of 100-millimetre height around the base of the portacot to allow good airflow and minimise the possibility of suffocation if baby snuggles against the side of the portacot.

Some states and territories in Australia have banned the sale and supply of some portable cots. Phone your local consumer affairs or fair trading office for information.

Before you buy

- Before you buy a new or second-hand portable cot, make sure that all locking devices are secure when the cot is assembled and that your child cannot release them and collapse the cot. Regularly check locking devices to ensure they are operating properly.
- If you are buying a second-hand portable cot, check there are no tears in the mesh or fabric sides and no cracks in the side rails. Also check that the portacot meets the latest safety standards and has a breathability zone around the base.

- Follow the assembly instructions closely when setting up the cot.
- Do not use a portable cot if your child weighs more than 15 kilograms.
- Do not put additional mattresses in a portable cot. Small children can become wedged between the mattress and soft sides of the cot and may suffocate. Older children may use the extra height to help them climb out.
- Check that all locking devices are properly latched before putting a child in the cot.
- Remove all toys from the cot when the child is sleeping.

The nursery

Comfort and calm

For many parents, planning and decorating a nursery can be akin to planning a flash wedding. Although preparing a space for your baby is one of the most joyous tasks of getting ready for welcoming a new little being, it is worth bearing in mind that you are doing this for yourself. Your baby may or may not seem impressed and your painstaking efforts may not influence his desire to sleep soundly, regardless of the designer cot or elegant nursery.

Whatever your family's sleeping arrangements, there are a few things to consider (besides safety) as you organise your baby's sleep space. As well as creating the best nest for your baby, consider your own needs too. For instance, you will be getting up to your baby at least for a few weeks or months so you might as well make this as pleasant and easy for yourself as possible. A comfy chair for night feeds or a safe space around your bed if you prefer to lie down and feed is essential. A small lamp or nightlight will allow you to do night feeds and nappy changes without turning on an overhead light (this may keep your baby from waking fully as you attend to him). A small CD player or iPod dock and a relaxing playlist or CDs will be calming and nurturing for you as well as your baby.

Is he too hot?

A typical late night discussion between parents tends to go along the lines of, 'Do you think he's too hot?' And the flipside, 'Do you think he's warm enough?'

It is a natural instinct to rug up your baby on cool winter nights but overheating is associated with an increased risk of SIDS, so it's important not to overdress your baby for bed. But babies and little children can also become too cold for comfort. A baby will sleep comfortably in a room heated to a temperature between sixteen and twenty degrees Celsius.

Your baby's hands and feet are not a good guide to how hot or cold he is – they often feel cold, yet your baby can be perfectly warm enough to sleep. Instead of feeling your baby's hands, check his core body temperature by placing your hand flat on the skin of your baby's chest or back to see that he is nice and warm, not too hot or cold.

If your baby is too hot, he will feel sweaty or clammy and may have a heat rash, especially around his neck, or he may look red in the face and cry. To cool him down, remove a layer of clothing or bedding. Often babies who are feeling cold become irritable and if your baby is too cold he may shiver, but a cold baby may also react by becoming still to try and conserve energy. Warm him up with a cuddle against your skin then add another layer of clothing and extra blankets.

Use your commonsense as you dress your baby for bed – if you feel warm enough wearing light pyjamas or a t-shirt to bed, your baby won't need to be rugged up in lots of layers with a wrap as well. If your baby is still swaddled, always use light clothing under the wrap and do not swaddle your baby if you are sharing a sleep surface. Do, though, consider how you feel trying to get to sleep with cold feet – accept all offers of bootees from grandma. You will need to keep baby's head uncovered to prevent overheating and please be sensitive to temperatures when you are out. If your baby is sleeping in his pram rugged up against the cold weather outdoors, and you pop into a heated shopping centre, you will need to remove a layer of clothing or you will soon have a grumpy, hot and possibly dehydrated baby.

An extra caution if you feel your baby has become hot and is thirsty – it is unsafe to give babies under six months water to drink, so either offer a breastfeed or formula. Giving water puts babies at greater risk for a serious condition called hyponatremia. When babies are given too much water, it dilutes the level of sodium in the blood. Sodium controls blood pressure and helps nerves and muscles work properly. Sodium is found in the body fluids outside the cells. If the sodium level is low, nearby cells take in water (swell) in an attempt to restore the balance. Brain cells are confined within the skull so when they swell, symptoms including hyponatremic seizures can occur resulting in brain damage or even death.

Natural fabric clothing and bedding is best for baby. Some babies can become uncomfortable and wakeful in response to irritation from synthetic materials. Take care, too, with laundry detergents, as some babies suffer from itching or snuffly noses due to perfumes and irritants in detergents.

Finally, make sure to turn clothing such as socks or jumpsuits inside out after washing to check for loose threads that can entrap tiny toes.

Decorations

When it comes to decorating a baby's room, there is a school of thought that advocates removing all stimulating objects such as toys and mobiles. I recently heard from a mother who had lovingly painted a picture for her baby's room. Her child health nurse had advised this mother to remove the picture as it would overstimulate the baby.

I find this advice pretty harsh and unnecessary: painting a picture or making a mobile for your baby is a lovely part of connecting even before you meet this new little person and the babies I know who do have mobiles often watch these as they wind down to sleep or as they wake up gradually. Watching mobiles (or leaves on a tree as baby sleeps outdoors) is a great eye-tracking exercise.

If you have an easily overstimulated baby, you can hang his mobiles above the change table so he can enjoy them when he is wide awake (and you need a distraction to entice him to keep still as you change him), rather than near his cot. Your newborn will lie with his head facing sideways at first in a pose rather like a fencer. This is due to an early reflex and will mean that he will be able to watch mobiles that hang beside him rather than over his head. In any case, it is safer not to have mobiles or pictures above your baby where they could possibly fall down and hurt him.

With an older baby, too many toys will probably cause overstimulation as your little one may have difficulty switching off from playtime, so a good storage cupboard or toybox is a useful addition to a child's room. Personally though, I love to see a baby's room that parents have put their heart and souls into, even if the baby will only use his room for playtime until he feels secure enough to sleep alone.

Black-out blinds

I have concerns about advice to use black-out blinds for daytime sleeps. While black-out blinds or dark curtains can be helpful to discourage early morning risers, babies' visual development is stimulated by natural light and movement, including the patterns sunlight creates as it flows into a room gently filtered by sheer curtains.

You can help your baby's visual development by moving his cot around or placing him in different places to sleep during the day, so he gets to look in all directions. This will help prevent flat spots on his head from always lying on the same side too. Having light flowing into a bedroom, or moving your baby's bedding around the house during the day will encourage your baby to develop a day–night sleep rhythm. Of course, if you have a baby who is extra sensitive, you may need to draw the curtains and create a quieter space for sleeps, but total blackness isn't necessary during the day.

Consider, too, how flexible you want your baby to be. Unless you are happy to stay at home indefinitely to accommodate all of your baby's sleeps, it is generally easier to have a baby who isn't accustomed to sleeping only in a dark room. Your baby needs sensory stimulation to help develop his nervous system – so he will ultimately sleep better as his nervous sytem matures. By sharing your normal daily activities with your baby – going for walks in the fresh air, visiting friends, or going to mum and baby classes such as yoga, swimming or baby gym, your baby will naturally become tired and sleep when and where he needs to. You will feel much better having your own social needs met too, rather than spending all day in a darkened room trying to make your baby sleep. Consider, don't you find it easier to relax and sleep better after time in the fresh air or after some exercise and social contact?

Having said this, I do understand that some babies and children are especially sensitive to sensory stimulation such as noise and light and it can be utter torment to these little people to be unable to shut it out. Some babies and small children with a low sensory threshold have responses to stimuli that can also affect their behaviour when they are awake.

The effects of sensory stimulation can be accumulative. For instance, some little ones will generally tolerate a reasonable level of stimulation but after exposure to a particularly noisy environment, they may become increasingly sensitive over the course of the day. Babies and children won't always react the same way and this can be confusing to parents who may think the child is being 'naughty'. In fact, sensitive babies and children are responding to a sensory overload and may find it difficult to tune out either when they are awake (and thus become 'hyperactive') or when it is time to sleep. You can help baby's immature nervous system by gradually increasing sensory input such as massage, gentle music and movement when she is awake – let her tolerance be your guide – or a sensory motor program such as GymbaROO.

So tune in to your individual baby and work his sleeping environment around his needs. As your little one's nervous system matures, he will gradually become more flexible. However, if he remains sensitive or you have any concerns about aspects of his development, seek advice from an appropriate health professional who can check for possible causes and offer help.

A child's view

When you set up your baby's sleeping space and when you move your toddler from a cot to a bed, consider things like draughts and noises (such as traffic or sounds from a television or computer through the wall). Consider what lights might shine in from outside or from the hallway in your home and how these lights may create shadows that will affect your child's sleep environment, especially at night-time. It can help to lie in the space in which you plan to place the cot or bed and see how it feels from the child's perspective because, just like us, little ones can be kept awake by annoying stimuli or discomfort.

Last but not least, a word on windows: make sure there are no dangling cords within reach of your child or near his cot and arrange furniture so a toddling tot can't get a leg up and out a window to make a silent getaway – it has happened!

6

Sharing sleep

'The bosom of a mother is the natural pillow of her offspring.'

Dr J T Conquest

Co-sleeping is not a guilty habit. I define co-sleeping as 'sleeping within sensory proximity to your infant' but also include the frequently taboo issue of bedsharing and its impact on bonding and sleep patterns. Despite research showing that between 50 to 80 per cent of parents share a bed with their infants at some time, or that breastfeeding and co-sleeping are inextricably linked, this option is often shrouded in secrecy or disapproval, not to mention outright fear-mongering: one advertising campaign in the US used images of a baby sleeping next to a large machete claiming this was as dangerous as a mother sleeping next to her infant!

When I have been speaking to groups of parents and asked, 'Is there anyone here who hasn't taken your baby into your bed to sleep – ever?' not a single hand has been raised in Australia, the US or New Zealand. Although this is certainly not a claim of research, it shows that sharing a bed with your baby is common enough that we have a duty of care to discuss bed sharing safety. An avoidance of discussion serves neither parents nor infants: it has simply resulted in a paucity of information about how to implement a safe sleep environment for infants who either occasionally or usually sleep with their parents.

> After having been to a mother and baby unit for two weeks and enduring the nightmare of trying to have my daughter and I 'conform' to controlled crying, I finally gave into what my instincts were telling me and returned to co-sleeping. My instincts must have been right, because one of the most memorable moments I have as a mother soon followed. Upon waking one sleepy Sunday morning, I was startled by some thing brushing close to my face. I opened my eyes wide, to find my beautiful baby daughter kneeling between my husband and I. She was facing me, leaning down and had planted the most sweet little kiss on my lips. It was the best thing I have ever woken up to and the memory of it is forever ingrained – something I will never forget. I was never so sure that this was what I was meant to be doing.
>
> Kelly

For any mother snuggling a baby, nuzzling her face into her infant's hair and smelling that sweet newborn breath, research to show that mothers and babies feel best when they are close to each other is about as necessary as research to show that grass will grow if it rains. That said, there is indeed scientific evidence that mothers and babies are hardwired to enjoy the experience of togetherness.

A mother's warm body next to a baby during the early months acts as a sort of 'pacemaker', somehow reminding the infant to breathe while her breathing and arousal mechanisms are immature. Your warm body can also help to keep your baby's temperature stable. For instance, a newborn has twice as much skin in proportion to his body size than an adult, and he loses heat much faster. Studies have shown that placing newborn infants on their mother's bare chest is more effective at maintaining the baby's body temperature than radiant heated cribs in delivery suites, even when their ambient temperatures were the same. A possible explanation for this loss of body heat in infants may be that a baby separated from its mother produces stress hormones such as cortisol, and these cause a drop in body temperature. Although over-heating is a concern (it is a potential SIDS risk factor), when baby and mother sleep in close contact and the baby is not overdressed, he will take on his mother's skin temperature so, if she becomes too hot, she can simply remove a layer of bedding.

Perhaps the strongest argument in favour of continuous mother-baby togetherness is that infants bond with their mother through all of their senses – eye contact, the sounds of their mother's voice, her touch and her smell. Attachment, the process of 'learning to love', is a behavioural system that does not deactivate during sleep and, as obstetrician Michel Odent observes, 'it takes only the most elementary observation to see that a baby needs its mother even more during the night than in the daylight. In the dark, the baby's predominant sense – sight – is at rest. Instead, the baby needs to use its sense of touch through skin-to-skin contact, and its sense of smell.'

> *People say they want to spend more time with their kids. Going to sleep and waking with a baby or small child is a wonderful way to bond in a natural way. Bedtime stress barely exists when kids know they will go to sleep and wake next to the most important people in their lives.*
>
> Danny

For parents who enjoy sharing sweet dreams with their baby, the research is affirming: touch and proximity are essential elements of bonding; the hormonal status that enhances bonding is at its most effective during night-time breastfeeding; continued breastfeeding maintains the release of hormones essential for mother–infant bonding, and breastfeeding is more likely to be successful for a longer duration when mothers and infants share sleep. Perhaps, without pressure to teach their babies as soon as possible to sleep all night, mothers could relax more and appreciate night-time breastfeeds as an extra opportunity to bond with their babies.

> *Elsbeth sleeps with us in our bed. Her cot has always been in our room. She has had times when she slept in her cot, although now she sleeps solely in our bed. In*

the early days, I remember struggling out of bed to pick her up during the night for feeding, which was made more difficult by a caesarean birth and wrist swelling from fluid retention when I was pregnant. I would prop myself up with pillows and feed for about an hour. Then I'd try diligently to settle her back to sleep in her cradle, as I'd been warned not to let her fall asleep on the breast or I would be making a rod for my back! I'd rock the cradle and sing lullabies over and over often for up to an hour. Eventually she'd fall asleep and then wake as I crept back into bed so we'd start the settling routine again.

Then sometimes I was so tired I would feed her lying down in our bed as I couldn't stay awake sitting up for an hour and she would fall asleep on the breast and I would fall asleep too. I'd wake several hours later for the next feed and again feed her lying down. Eventually, we were both sleeping for ten to twelve hours each night, minus the time to feed, and we haven't looked back.

I get really annoyed when I think about the advice I received from the hospital, early childhood centre and in brochures from sleep training centres that it's wrong to feed your baby to sleep or to have your baby in bed with you. How could something that feels so right and actually works be wrong? When going down the other track, I was overtired, my baby was overtired, we were both stressed and I could well and truly feel a rod digging into my back!

Kimberley

There are risk factors to be aware of for formula-feeding mothers who are considering sharing a bed with their baby: video footage from baby sleep labs at Durham University, UK, and the University of Notre Dame, Indiana, show that breastfeeding, bedsharing mothers intuitively create a protective space around their babies by lying on their side, with baby in the crook of their arm or with the mother's lower arm bent upwards and knees bent, preventing baby from slipping down in the bed. This prevents the mother rolling towards her baby and means her partner can't roll into that protected space. Breastfed babies instinctively snuggle towards mum's breast, away from pillows that could potentially be a suffocation hazard. Conversely, formula-feeding mothers were more likely to hold babies up on the pillow or turn their backs on their babies while bedsharing.

If you are not breastfeeding, you can still work with an awareness of hormonal connections to bond with your baby through skin contact, such as bathing together and infant massage. Eye contact with your baby releases endorphins in both your bodies and this too is an important element of bonding.

I have had a number of women attending my classes who, because of traumatic birth experiences and early separation or improper advice, have experienced insurmountable breastfeeding difficulties. Some of these mothers expressed a sense of despair and desperation to bond with their babies, so made conscious choices to learn baby massage and to sleep with their babies in close proximity in a separate safe sleep space such as a co-sleeper cot attached to the parents' bed. From my observations, touch is an extremely powerful bonding tool and within a couple of weeks of skin-to-skin contact – bathing with their babies, massage and cuddling their sleeping babies during the day, mothers and babies are soon closely connected, regardless of their sleeping arrangements or whether they are breastfed.

> *The whole co-sleeping arrangement suits all of us. We don't have to get out of bed and walk to another room – if he wakes up we just have a cuddle and then it's back to sleep for us all. When my son was small and still having regular bottles . . . we had a bottle with warm water inside a foam bottle warmer, and a formula dispenser next to it on the nightstand. When he needed a drink all we had to do was mix the two together, wait for him to finish his milk, cuddle him back to sleep then place him in his co-sleeper cot right next to us. Who says you have to get out of bed?*
>
> **Leah**

Three is not a crowd

The notion of a family bed may have absolutely no appeal to you. However, before you argue, 'our baby will *never* sleep in our bed', please consider that in one study at Adelaide University, more than 80 per cent of parents had taken their babies into their bed at some time. Two larger studies in the UK found that almost half of all newborns bedshared at some time with their parents and on any one night in the first month over a quarter of parents slept with their baby. When considering common factors that may influence bedsharing, researchers found no relation between warmer months, colder months, weekends, age or marital status of mothers or socio-economic status of families. In fact, bedsharing was more common among the least deprived during the first months of life and was strongly associated with breastfeeding.

> I don't recall when and how my partner first broached the topic of co-sleeping. I believe my first reaction was that it sounded quite natural and commonsense. However, at the time, I did not fully understand the impact it would have on me as a father and as a part-ner, and also the effect it would have on the bond we have as a family.
>
> As we are now coming up to our fourth year of co-sleeping, with our eldest having recently moved into his own bed in his own room, I realise it has been a wonderful, nurturing experience. I feel as a dad, working long hours away from the family home, that spending time asleep with my kids has been invaluable, especially to help me to create a closer connection individually, and as a family.
>
> I treasure the numerous moments over the years of waking up in the middle of the night to the sound of a small, quiet breath next to me. Of waking up to realise that I and my son had been sleeping face to face not inches away from each other, or that I had been sleeping

in the nook of his armpit for a part of the night!

I firmly believe it has had innumerable benefits for all of us, especially the children. I myself could think of nothing better than being small, in my parents' bed, all warm, snug, cosy and safe on a cold, dark and scary night. It has made them feel important, loved and cared for, and I see it in their expression when they wake up in the morning next to us – the twinkle in their eye, the smile on their face and the look of joy and love.

Adam

According to Professor James McKenna, 'Co-sleeping is a safe and even potentially life-saving option, as long as parents provide a safe sleeping environment.' Professor McKenna has extensively studied mothers and babies both co-sleeping and sleeping separately, and his research demonstrates what some co-sleeping mothers will attest that when mothers and babies sleep together, they tend to get into the same sleep cycle. The mothers, even in deep sleep, were aware of their babies' positions and would move to avoid lying on them or impeding their breathing. Although the co-sleeping babies spent less time in deep sleep and aroused more frequently (though not necessarily waking), their mothers actually got *more* sleep than the mother–baby pairs sleeping in separate rooms.

As a researcher in SIDS, Professor McKenna explains that these small transient arousals may lessen a baby's susceptibility to some forms of SIDS which are thought to be caused by failure to arouse from deep sleep to re-establish breathing patterns. The babies in his studies who sleep with their mothers also tend to sleep on their backs or sides and less often on their tummies, another factor that could reduce the risk of SIDS. Professor McKenna advises, 'From an evolutionary and biological perspective, proximity to parental sounds, smells, gases, heat and movement during the night is precisely what the human infant "expects", and in our push for infant independence, we are forgetting that an infant's biology cannot change quite as quickly as cultural child-care patterns.'

Ironically, it was concern about this very proximity to parental 'gasses' that resulted in caution against co-sleeping for babies of the Victorian era. An 1888 article in *Baby*, a pioneer of today's baby magazines, advises, 'for the first few weeks, animal heat is usually maintained by sleeping with the mother, but on no account should a child of later age sleep between two persons, as by doing so it must of necessity breathe the emanations from their bodies.'

A conspiracy of silence

Publicity over recent years has raised doubts about the safety of bedsharing with infants. Opponents of co-sleeping present the image of a mother's body as no more responsive than an inert cot mattress or at worst, as dangerous as a large machete. This undermining of a mother's confidence in her ability to nurture and protect her baby is hardly conducive to enhanced mother–infant bonding and, I believe, may increase any potential risks due to unsafe co-sleeping as mothers go 'underground' about sleeping with their babies.

Diana West, US lactation consultant and co-author of *Sweet Sleep, Nighttime and Naptime Strategies for the Breast-fed Baby* says, '"Never Bedshare" sounds great on paper (or billboards). But the public health agencies promoting it forget that babies need to be fed at night. And they don't take into account that breastfeeding releases hormones that makes mothers feel sleepy during the feeding. So where are mothers supposed to breastfeed their babies at night? They never say. Mothers are left struggling to find a place to feed the baby where they can doze during the nursing. Thinking that it's too dangerous to bring the baby into their own bed, research has shown that almost half of mothers sleep with their babies on sofas, upholstered chairs, or recliners at some point. But that's an incredibly risky place for suffocation because of all the crevices and padding.'

> I have lovely memories of sleeping with my parents when I was little. I also remember comments from friends when my youngest brother was born while I was completing my final year at secondary school. People would say, 'It must be hard to study with a baby in the house,' but I wasn't woken by my brother because he slept with our parents, so he never had to cry in the night.
>
> It wasn't until I was studying midwifery that I realised sleeping with infants was unusual and that some maternity hospitals even had a policy against allowing babies in their mother's beds.
>
> **Kate, midwife**

While I am not necessarily advocating that you should share a bed with your baby – that decision is yours – I feel it is responsible to be realistic that, like so many parents, there is a likelihood that you will at some stage either sneak your baby into your bed in the desperate hope of a few hours sleep, or you and your partner may make a conscious decision to co-sleep.

> On our first night home from hospital, I handed Marisa to my partner as I got her cot ready. John was cuddling her in our bed and they looked so beautiful together that I went off to find the camera. By the time I got back, they were both sound asleep. I was so exhausted that, rather than risk disturbing them, I just got into bed and we all slept snuggled up together.
>
> I learned very quickly that sleeping with your baby was definitely against the rules. Marisa was sleeping well in bed with us but I kept thinking she wasn't supposed to be there. I was in information overload and, depending on what I read or who had made negative comments, I swung between sleeping with Marisa, and putting her in her cot. Eventually, after failing a stint at sleep school and lots of crying, through sheer exhaustion, I took her back into our bed. We all relaxed and slept again, and Marisa became happy during the day too.
>
> Kelly

It is normal for breastfed babies to feed frequently and for long periods in the first few weeks after delivery. Breastfeeding hormones have a soporific effect on you as well as your baby – this is nature's way of ensuring you get plenty of rest so you recover after the enormous task of growing and birthing a baby. Whether you are breast- or bottle-feeding, if you choose not to take your baby into your bed, be aware there is a potential risk that as you sit feeding your baby on a sofa or chair, you could fall asleep and possibly drop your baby or end up in an unsafe position. There is also a chance that the sleep deprivation caused by sitting up for large parts of the night will drive you to either ignore safety recommendations and take your baby into bed when you are excessively tired (a known SIDS risk factor since your awareness and responsiveness are reduced) or to give up breastfeeding.

Safe co-sleeping

Whatever your sleeping arrangements, it is important to provide a safe sleeping environment for your baby. If you choose to sleep with your baby, both parents should feel comfortable with the decision and accept equal responsibility. For some parents, co-sleeping will not be appropriate, particularly if one of you is on medication that affects your awareness, is a heavy snorer or has sleep apnoea, or if you have an extremely restless baby. Since adult beds are not designed with infant safety in mind, it is sensible to take some basic precautions.

Maternal-infant sleep researchers have found that there are seven main risk factors for SIDS and suffocation:

1. Adult smoking
2. A caregiver under the influence of alcohol or other sedatives
3. Formula-feeding
4. A baby with a health problem that prevents normal arousal from sleep
5. Baby sleeping on his stomach
6. An overheated baby
7. A baby sleeping on a surface with gaps, crevices, or pillowy objects.

La Leche League International, the world's oldest and largest volunteer breastfeeding organisation, calls these seven bedsharing risk factors The Safe Sleep Seven. If a breastfeeding mother doesn't smoke or go to bed sedated, and her healthy, not overdressed baby is sleeping by her side on his back on a safe surface, then she and her baby meet The Safe Sleep Seven and baby is at extremely low risk for either SIDS or suffocation. Even the researchers who warn against bedsharing agree that by about four months, bedsharing by any responsible, nonsmoking adult is as safe as having your baby sleep separately in a bassinette or crib.

Diana West advises, 'teaching parents about The Safe Sleep Seven and how to make their bed surface safe for bedsharing is a helpful tool to help parents understand the real risks and protect babies from SIDS and suffocation. This is true even if they don't ever plan to bedshare, because a pre-planned bed is much safer than a sofa or recliner. It is simple childproofing. Most parents go to great lengths to protect outlets and cabinets because they know accidents can happen, no matter how watchful they are. Not every mother and baby can bedshare safely, but it's still safer to for every mother to make her bed as safe as possible just in case.'

Other precautions to consider include:

- If you have long hair, tie it back, remove jewellery and avoid clothes with string ties. If you are obese or large-breasted, consider that you may not be able to feel exactly where your infant is. Having said this, I doubt there is an unsafe weight per se, but that the safety of your baby depends on your own body awareness.

- Take precautions to prevent baby from rolling out of bed. Perhaps place the bed against a wall or on the floor or use guardrails. Don't leave a baby on an adult bed unattended. This doesn't mean you have to go to bed at the same time as your baby every night. You can settle her in a cot until you go to bed or until she wakes, then transfer her into your bed.

- The sleeping surface should be clean and firm (waterbeds and sofas are unsafe and pillow top mattresses should also be regarded with caution), the mattress should tightly intersect the bed frame, and your baby's head should never be covered.

Making co-sleeping work

Co-sleeping defines a range of options, including bed-sharing, but generally means mother and baby sleep within sensory reach of each other. It can include a cradle, cot or hammock next to your bed or taking your baby into your bed with you.

Bedsharing can encompass a range of creative set-ups: some babies sleep on their own small mattress above and between the parents in the adult bed; some parents choose to remove a cot-side and butt the baby's cot against their bed. If you do this, make sure there are no gaps for your baby to slip into and that the cot is safely positioned so it can't roll away from the bed – securely tucking a sheet across your mattress and the baby's mattress is one option for eliminating a potential gap.

Some parents turn their bed sideways, sacrificing length for a few inches of extra width. Others put two beds together – parents of twins explained how they stitched sheets together to fit across a queen bed and a single bed pushed together. Other families move their mattress onto the floor, which is especially good if their baby sleeps in the adult bed during the day. Of course, the surrounding space must also be safe and/or a door gate used in case baby wakes unattended.

All of the children slept in our bed for between one and three years. Ella being the first didn't even have her own bedroom till she was two. It was kind of a treat to set it up and encourage her to start to move out of our bed. Generally what would happen is that she would start in her room and then come back to ours later in the night. We never pushed the issue and always let her decide what she wanted to do. People are a bit shocked when they realise I don't have a nursery for the babies. I always think what a waste of a room!

Paul and I have also been flexible with musical beds. If a child was sick, one of us would move in with them. If someone was lonely and there was already someone else in our bed one of the adults would go to the kids' bed. That is the beauty of having more than one double bed in the house.

Maxine

Sleeping with your baby doesn't have to be an all-or-nothing proposition, nor does it mean you have to go to bed at the same time as your baby every night. Despite the convenience of not having to get out of bed and the delight of snuggling with your baby, it is very natural to feel all touched out after caring for a baby all day or you may be too exhausted during the first part of the night to be fully responsive to your baby if she is in bed with you.

It is also perfectly normal to want to reclaim your body or your partner's body. (Mind you, you can employ creativity here – you don't only have to make love in bed, at night!) Some parents start off with their baby sleeping in his own bed and bring him into their bed when he wakes, others take their baby into their bed for an early morning cuddle, some mothers enjoy co-sleeping or dozing and breastfeeding during an afternoon siesta.

I found that our newborn daughter would settle into her cradle most nights, but after waking for a feed, she would have difficulty settling back to bed. I would then pop her into bed with us and she would sleep well. We would continue our feeds lying down which I found very comfortable as I was experiencing a lot of upper back pain from feeding.

Kim

Matilda co-slept with us from minute one . . . We co-slept until she was ten weeks when she refused to sleep near us, so she went into a cot at the base of the bed and would sleep there until early morning and then join us. At six months Matilda moved into her own cot and slept heaps better on her own.

From that day onwards, whenever we brought her into our room for a family sleep, she refused and will not sleep with us in the bed with her. I was very sad because I felt like I lost contact with her. Now at eleven months I realise that a huge part of her personality is being independent and it makes sense, but I was pretty upset over it. She had one sleep alone in her bed and that was it, no going back.

Christy

Getting comfortable

Just as it took you a while to adapt to sleeping with your partner, sharing a bed with your baby will probably take a little while to get used to. (Even sharing a room with your baby can take some getting used to as you are aware of every little sniffle and grunt.) At first you will be very aware of your baby's presence but as you get used to sharing sleep, you will stop worrying about what your baby is doing as she sleeps. In case this sounds a little scary to you, consider when the last time was that you fell out of bed. Or lost your pillow. Just as you know exactly where the edge of the bed is when you sleep, you will be aware of your baby, too, provided you are healthy, sober and unmedicated.

Although you will find your own way to feel comfortable and safe with your baby snuggled next to you, if you do bedshare, as has been shown to be intuitive for breastfeeding mothers, I would suggest sleeping on your side with your knees bent below your baby and your baby tucked in the crook of your elbow with his head resting on your arm or your lower arm facing upwards, above your baby's head. Although when my own babies were young, there was no scientific evidence that this was natural and safe, I felt safe this way: I couldn't roll over an outstretched arm and I felt aware of where my baby was, rather than having him or her loose in the bed between myself and my partner or on the edge of the bed.

Science now affirms that this 'cuddle cove' is not only instinctive to all mammals (note how a cat sleeps curled around her kittens), but it forms a protective space around your sleeping baby – your baby will be sleeping on his back, you won't be able to roll over without arousing yourself and if your partner is in the bed, they won't be able to accidentally roll onto your baby. Meanwhile, your knees bent below your baby will prevent him from sliding beneath bed covers.

Breastfeeding will be easier with your baby next to you – you simply feel your baby rooting and latch him on before either of you are wide awake. This saves so much time resettling a baby who has woken completely because you have had to get up before responding. After the early months a baby can usually 'help himself' and because you and your baby will share sleep cycles you won't be woken from a deep sleep as your baby stirs, then find yourself wide awake and unable to get back to sleep easily after you have fed him.

You don't need to worry too much which breast your baby had last. You will find yourself rolling your baby across you onto your other arm as you change sides for sleeping comfort, so she will get both breasts during the night if she wakes to feed. If you are a bit lopsided in the morning, give her the 'big' breast for breakfast.

From bed to bed

If you are co-sleeping and facing criticism ('you will never get him out of your bed!') or concerned about creating bad habits, take heart. In a study from the University of California, researchers looking at the correspondence between sleeping arrangements and independence found that although solitary sleeping children fell asleep alone and slept through the night at an earlier age, early co-sleepers were the most self-reliant preschoolers. For example, these children exhibited behaviours such as getting dressed without help and entertaining themselves with a book or toy. Early co-sleepers also demonstrated the most independence with their peers: they were more likely to initiate friendships and work out problems with playmates.

As you make any changes, it is wise to remember the mantra 'gradually with love' and make each change in baby steps. For instance, you might move your baby from your bed to a cot next to your bed; later you might move the cot to the other side of your room. Your baby or toddler may have day sleeps in her cot or bed, then as she feels secure and associates her own bed with sleep times, you can include night sleeps there too or you might move your child from your bed straight into a single bed or, if you are worried about falls, a single bed mattress on the floor where, if you need to offer comfort at night, you can snuggle in your child's bed, depending on her age at the time of transition. Toddlers who are old enough to talk (around two or older) often love the fuss of shopping for a new doona and sleeping in their own 'big person' bed; however, you may wish to move your baby out of your bed sooner. Some toddlers who are bedsharing and breast-feeding can become 'all night suckers' and a little distance from the breast can encourage longer sleeps – just think how enticing it would be for you to nibble all night if you slept with a delicious chocolate muffin on your pillow!

If you take each step as you and your child are ready, then change is likely to be more permanent, although it is natural for little backward steps at times of stress or sickness. If you pressure your baby into making changes that he isn't ready for, the trade-off could be whiny, clingy behaviour or broken sleep.

One of the advantages that I have noticed with my own children, who shared our bed for varying lengths of time and frequency, was that they never went through the so-called normal stages that are described in many child-care books and magazines, such as having a transitional object or a 'lovey', head-banging in their cots, 'bedtime battles' or fear of the dark. It was only when my third child was about three years old that I realised my children had completely missed these stages. She would get up in the night and take herself to the toilet then patter back to her bed or wriggle in with us some nights without calling out or disturbing us. Although it hadn't previously occurred to me, this absence of fear of the dark made sense for her (as it had for her older brothers) because she never had to associate night-time with being left alone.

Caitlin is four years old and sleeps in her bed most nights. Occasionally she will come into our bed and we cuddle for a while and then I take her back to her room where she peacefully sleeps till morning. Madeleine is now eighteen months old and transitioned from our bed to hers with no drama whatsoever. She was an active baby in her sleep and was waking herself so she moved to a single bed at about twelve months. She wakes in the morning, grabs her pillow and comes in to wake mummy with her gorgeous smile, followed shortly by

Caitlin . . . then there is four in the bed till we all rise
(sometimes I think a king-sized bed would help). I think
the reassurance that they are always able to get a cuddle when they want has helped my daughters become
independent toddlers and young children.

I am hoping they will still visit our beds until they move
out of home as this is always a secure place for special
chats and the creation of a lifelong tradition that I am
hoping will help me cope with teenagers.

Lisa

I have co-slept with two of my babies and we are in
the process of weaning off those wonderful night-time
snuggles. Eva has slept with us, either in a cradle,
pushed close to the bed or between us since she first
came home. I packed the cot away when I realised that
I had no desire to put her to sleep in it. Everyone slept
so well when she slept with us.

She is nearly three now and has become an
inconsiderate bed partner. She has taken to sleeping
in the H-position (feet on one parent, head on the
other!) and I have the growing feeling that this is
because she needs more space. The time has come.
I will miss her cheek pushed up next to mine and the
sweet milky smell of her breath. I will also miss gazing
at her peaceful sleeping face in the pre-dawn light. My
grandmother (after whom Eva is named) used to tell
me that sleeping children look so peaceful because they
are gazing at angels. Surely she was right.

Now the time has come I am excited that Eva

is facing her next big adventure. We went shopping together and bought a small mattress and pillow. I went out on my own and bought her a little present. We put the mattress beside the bed and made it up so it looks very cosy. Eva even practised going to sleep there. We talked about everyone sleeping in their own space – big brothers Jack and Noah, even the birds in the trees – and I told her that after she fell asleep I would put her on her own pillow for the night. I also showed her that I would be close by if she needed a cuddle. We talked about the morning fairy. If Eva stayed on her own pillow until morning, three nights in a row, the morning fairy would bring her a special gift.

After mummy-milk, teeth and story time, Eva fell asleep in our bed as usual and I picked her up and placed her on the mattress by the bed. When she woke in the small hours, she climbed into mummy-bed for a cuddle and there she stayed until the boys joined us at daybreak.

The next couple of nights she woke earlier and earlier for her mummy-cuddle. She's a bright little thing and I got the feeling I was being scammed – and she still seemed to want the lion's share of the bed. Time to get a bit tougher.

When she woke that night and asked to come into bed, I told her she could have a cuddle on her pillow and then she would have to go back to sleep there. She was okay with that until I returned to my bed. She cried and she stamped her foot. I played possum. She walked around to her daddy's side of the bed. She cried. He

said, 'Time to go back to sleep on your very own pillow.'
She stamped her feet and I felt sure she would wake the
rest of the house. We played possum. Within moments
she had returned to her little mattress by the bed.
I leaned down and covered her up. The morning fairy
visited three days later.

We will slowly move her mattress towards the door,
into her own room and then she'll move into her own
bed. But you know what? I'm not ready.

Nina

7

Feed me

'The newborn baby will have only three demands. They are warmth in the arms of its mother, food from her breasts, and security in the knowledge of her presence. Breastfeeding satisfies all three.'

Dr Grantly Dick-Read

If you have a baby who sleeps for short periods during the day or wakes more than normal during the night (the definition of normal depends who is offering advice), you can be certain to be questioned or advised about your feeding schedule. Some people will say that you are not following a prescribed feeding schedule correctly or that you have been inconsistent in implementing a routine or that you have created your baby's feeding and sleeping problems. Others – even perfect strangers – may advocate such remedies as complementary formula or a bowl of cereal before bed and even stretching out your baby's feed times, perhaps by using a dummy, so your breasts fill up with milk. No matter how desperate you are for sleep, please don't try *any* of these suggestions before reading this chapter. Such advice is utterly at odds with healthy infant feeding practices and is unlikely to achieve your aim of a sleeping baby.

Breast or bottle?

Research affirms that your own milk will meet your baby's complex nutritional and immunological needs in ways that can't be duplicated by artificial substitutes. Human breastmilk is a living fluid containing organisms and proteins that offer protection against bacteria and viruses: if you catch a bug, specialised white blood cells will appear in your breastmilk to protect your baby and, conversely, if your baby becomes sick, the transfer of germs from baby's saliva to your breast will trigger the production of specific antibodies. Breastfeeding also aids your baby's speech, eyesight and intelligence and promotes a special bond between you and your baby. Formula feeding can increase the risk of your baby suffering from acute diarrhoea, respiratory, urinary tract and ear infections, asthma and allergies, coeliac disease, ulcerative colitis, insulin dependent diabetes and childhood lymphomas. As your baby grows, the composition of your breastmilk changes, to meet her changing needs. Some immune compounds in breastmilk have been shown to increase at about six months (just when babies become mobile and are exposed to a greater range of germs) and, in many instances, the long-term protective effects of breastfeeding are related to its duration.

Apart from a healthy baby, the benefits for mothers who breastfeed include less postpartum bleeding, delayed return of menstruation after childbirth, a reduced incidence of obesity later in life, and protection against osteoporosis, ovarian cancer and pre-menopausal breast cancer. Of course, the more obvious benefits include the convenience of no dirty dishes or bottles to wash or prepare in the dead of night.

It is generally true that breastfed babies will be more active and sleep less than formula-fed babies: they tend to sit, crawl and stand earlier and bouts of sleep tend to be shorter because breastfed babies need to be fed more frequently. (Your breastmilk is more easily digested than formula, which is based on cow's milk.) In the second half of the first year, breastfed babies will sleep less than formula-fed babies: in one study where mothers kept diaries, formula-fed babies at thirteen months were sleeping an average of fourteen hours, while breastfed babies were sleeping eleven hours out of twenty-four.

While this can come as a relief (or not) if you are breastfeeding and have been comparing your baby's sleep patterns with a friend's formula-fed baby and wondering what you are doing wrong, it is not a good reason to wean your baby or to offer bottles of formula in the hope that your baby will sleep more. This extra activity and learning time is a bonus to your baby's development, and the trade-off of trying to zonk your baby with formula could actually be a more wakeful or cranky baby due to health problems such as allergies, coughs and colds or ear infections. This is especially important to consider with a very young baby whose immature gut and immune system make him more vulnerable to illness or discomfort from symptoms such as tummy upsets or constipation, even after a single bottle of formula.

Although breastfeeding is a natural process, it doesn't always come easily so it is wise to find out as much as you can about breastfeeding before you are pacing the floor with a wakeful, unsettled baby. Attend some meetings at your local Australian Breastfeeding Association or La Leche League group, where you will get to know the people who can help you if you have difficulties. Read a good breastfeeding book and keep it handy when you have your baby so you can dispel conflicting information. Try *Breastfeeding . . . Naturally* by the Australian Breastfeeding Association, *The Womanly Art of Breastfeeding* by the La Leche League or, for basic breastfeeding and practical baby care information, see my book *Parenting by Heart*.

If you are bottle-feeding either formula or expressed breastmilk you can, of course, bond with your baby and offer beautiful nurturing with lots of skin contact and cuddles.

Remember to change sides so baby receives stimulation to both sides of his body. If you are feeling sad about weaning, your feelings are perfectly normal. It is natural to mourn the loss of a breastfeeding relationship and depending on why and how this ended, you may also feel angry and cheated if it was due to factors beyond your control.

Something that is seldom acknowledged is a 'weaning depression' due to the physiological effects of withdrawal from breastfeeding hormones. If this seems to be happening and you are having mood swings and teariness lasting more than a couple of weeks, please seek medical help. In any case if you are feeling sad about weaning before you felt ready, be kind to yourself and try to find somebody who will really listen to you without minimising your experience. Remember too, *every* breastfeed is a success: no matter how long you breastfeed – whether this is for one feed, one week, a month, a year or longer – or how much breastmilk you are able to give your baby, this magic potion is like medicine for your baby.

It's not just about the milk

Feeding your baby by bottle or breast is not simply a matter of giving him optimum nutrition or seeing that he drinks enough milk. When you are expected to time how many minutes you breastfeed, watch the hours between feeds or count how many feeds your baby has in a day, with the ultimate goal being how many hours you can make your baby sleep, you will soon see feeding your baby as a chore, or one more thing that you have to do, over and over. As resentment brews about how much time your baby is taking up, it can seem an attractive option to prop your baby with a bottle in the hope that your life will become more efficient.

I would like to offer another perspective: feeding your

baby is about much more than milk. In the early months, feeding will take more time and your baby will need to feed often. However, whether bottle- or breastfeeding, try to see this time as an expression of your love for your baby. In doing so, you will be able to appreciate the rewards of these intimate moments – breathing in your baby's delicious smell, stroking his silky skin as his warm little body snuggles against your own, and gazing into his trusting eyes as they meet yours – and you will cherish this precious time long after he has outgrown your lap.

Bottle-feeding, whether you are giving your baby formula or expressed breastmilk, can be as time-consuming as breastfeeding, especially if your baby feeds slowly as some very little babies do. The solution to a slow or sleepy feeding baby is not to force him to stay awake by brutal means such as sponging him with wet face washers (I kid you not, I have seen this advised) or by cutting a bigger hole in the teat – this poses a choking risk and most certainly would cause discomfort and distress. Rather, follow your baby's lead and perhaps offer smaller, more frequent feeds. As he grows stronger, he will find it easier to stay awake and will become a more efficient feeder naturally.

Above all, if you can see feeding your baby as a loving relationship, not a measure of how much milk you can get into him, your baby will feed better because he isn't feeling stressed at feed times and he will absorb the nutrients in his food more efficiently. He will also develop a healthy association with feeding that is likely to be reflected in a smooth transition to solid foods when he is ready, and healthy eating habits as he grows.

How often should I feed my baby?

It can feel very reassuring to have specific instructions about when to feed your baby, especially when everything about caring for a baby is new and uncertain to you. It is better, though, to learn how to read your individual baby's hunger cues and feed her when she is hungry or thirsty (just as you would eat and drink yourself). This may sound difficult but, despite claims by various people that a feeding schedule will positively influence your baby's sleep patterns, in most cases there are risks to be considered: some strict regimes have been associated with breastmilk supply failure, poor infant weight gain and failing to thrive infants.

There is also evidence that allowing babies to feed according to their own appetite, rather than imposing feeding schedules, is more compatible with the biology of mothers and babies. Although breastfeeding according to a schedule may seem to work at first, many women who use strict feeding schedules in the early weeks find that their milk supply dwindles and their baby may be weaned by about three months. By restricting feeds or repeatedly spacing them out with dummies, you may limit the development of the hormonal process that enhances ongoing milk production. In the early days, your breasts need frequent stimulation to 'set' your milk production capacity as your milk supply is influenced by post-birth hormones. Also, in the first three months after birth, there is more breast development happening – you are developing more prolactin receptors, which will encourage your ongoing milk supply. Early and frequent breastfeeding will promote a continuing milk supply, which means that your baby will get lots of milk so he is less likely to wake up often to be fed.

The amount of breastmilk you produce and how much your baby drinks is influenced by factors including your baby's stomach size and the milk storage capacity of your own breasts. At first, your baby's tummy is only the size of his tiny fist and breastmilk is very quickly digested so your baby will need frequent feeds, at least in the early weeks. It is common for a breastfed baby to need feeding from several times in one hour to about every two hours at first – and that means two hours from the beginning of one feed to the beginning of the next, not two hours between feeds. It is also common for babies to need a cluster of feeds closer together in the evening.

Ultrasound studies by biochemist Dr Peter Hartmann and colleagues at the University of Western Australia have shown that breastmilk storage capacity can vary up to three times as much between individual women (this is not necessarily related to breast size and doesn't influence *milk production* ability). This means that while some women who have a large milk storage capacity will be able to feed their babies enough milk to go three or four hours between feeds (providing their baby has a big enough stomach), other women will need to feed their babies more often. For women with a smaller milk storage capacity, a three- or four-hourly feeding schedule could result in a hungry, unsettled baby and a mother who questions her ability to produce enough milk when really, it is the schedule that is inappropriate, not the mother's feeding ability. Instead of becoming stressed about how much milk your breasts are making or storing, think in terms of drinking out of a cup – you can still drink a litre of water whether you drink it from a large cup or several small cupfuls. If you allow your baby to nurse whenever he lets you know he is hungry, you will never have to worry about your milk storage capacity.

Milk production and infant intake are also influenced by the fat content of your milk and the degree of breast emptying at any given feeding. According to Dr Hartmann's research, an empty breast will make milk more quickly while a full breast will make milk more slowly. This means that milk production will speed up or slow down according to how hungry your baby is and how well he empties your breasts – if he sucks vigorously and empties the breast (because you make milk continuously your breasts will never be completely empty), production speeds up, and if he doesn't take much milk from the breast at a feeding, your breasts will get the message to make less milk. If your baby seems to go on a feeding binge at any time, this isn't an indicator that you will lose your milk but that you will need to take it easy and feed your baby more frequently for a few days so your breasts get the message to produce more milk. By responding to your baby's signals, in a few days' time he will space out his feeds again.

Babies also regulate the type of milk they need by the way they suck. The first type, the foremilk, will quench their thirst, which is why they often have short, frequent feeds on hot days, just as we sip from our water bottles. Hunger will be satisfied by longer sucking periods when baby gets the fatty hindmilk, which is squeezed down into your ducts by the reflex known as 'letdown': this is usually felt as a tingly sensation in your breasts and accompanied by leaking from the breast that your baby is not sucking from. Letting your baby decide how long he needs to feed and letting him finish the first breast before switching sides, rather than limiting him to an arbitrary number of minutes each side, will ensure he gets the rich, fatty hindmilk.

There will be times when your baby has a growth spurt and will need to feed more often to match his increasing appetite. Babies who are unwell also often increase their feeding frequency. Researchers now believe that this not only provides comfort, but also increases the baby's intake of antibodies and immune factors through the mother's breastmilk.

So, it is better to watch your baby, not the clock, because if your baby is hungry but is not allowed to breastfeed, your breasts will remain full and your milk production will slow down. Also, if you offer a bottle as a top-up, your baby won't be sucking the whole amount of milk from your breasts so they won't get the message to produce the amount of milk he needs. As you offer another bottle, and so on, the decreased sucking will cause your milk supply to dwindle until soon your baby will be refusing your low milk supply in favour of a fast-flowing bottle and, before you realise, he will be weaned.

Do I have enough milk?

Some sleep specialists or health workers may suggest that your baby's wakefulness or failure to adhere to a regimented feeding regime is due to low breastmilk supply and may suggest you do a yield by expressing and measuring how much breastmilk you are producing. Whatever amount of milk you express, this is no indicator of how much an efficiently sucking baby will get. Besides, the performance anxiety of expressing to measure your milk quantity is enough to inhibit the letdown reflex which makes your milk flow. It is also important to be aware that a baby needs to drink larger quantities of formula to get adequate nutrition in comparison to breastmilk: you don't need to give your baby the same quantity of breastmilk as formula feeding charts will say a baby should drink at each feed. Also, measuring the quantity of expressed milk will not allow for the varying amounts of fat in your milk and this is the important factor. It is the fats in breastmilk that cause your baby to feel satisfied and help him sleep longer between feeds.

While there are certain medical conditions that may create challenges to breastmilk supply, such as PCOS, diabetes, thyroid disorders, low iron levels, high blood pressure and a condition called insufficient glandular tissue (red flags include a lack of breast development during puberty and pregnancy and/or tubular shaped breasts that are widely spaced), there are also a lot of 'booby traps' that have mothers reaching for the bottle when what they are experiencing is perfectly normal or can be fixed quite simply with the right advice and support.

If you are having a hard time, you don't need to ditch your nursing bra just yet. Try to remember, whether you can exclusively breastfeed or not, every drop of mummy-milk is liquid gold and there is help available. Calling in an expert such as an International Board Certified Lactation Consultant could make a world of difference to your confidence and your breastfeeding experience.

Now let's bust some typical booby traps around low milk supply.

My baby feeds all the time

Your newborn's stomach is the size of a marble and after about ten days it will only be the size of his tiny fist (or a ping pong ball if you don't yet have a baby and can't visualise this), so he will need frequent feeds – around eight to twelve feeds in twenty-four hours. Also, in the early weeks your baby is mastering the art of sucking, swallowing and breathing so he needs lots of practice to become an efficient feeder. It's also worth understanding that women have different breastmilk storage capacities so although most women produce enough milk, a woman with a smaller storage capacity (this isn't necessarily related to breast size) will need to feed her baby more often than a woman with a larger storage capacity, whatever the age of the baby.

Tip: watch your baby, not the clock. In the early weeks breast development is still occurring and by feeding according to your baby's hunger cues, you are setting your breasts' capacity for milk production. But if you space out feeds (by implementing a feeding schedule) or top your baby up with formula, she naturally eats less at the breast and your breasts will respond by making less milk. If you do need to offer supplements (first rule is 'feed the baby'), expressing, as well as putting your baby to the breast, will help increase your supply.

My breasts feel soft

At first your breasts will feel hard and swollen as your milk comes in but a lot of the swelling (engorgement) is extra blood circulation and tissue fluid as your body gets used to this new experience. As your baby and your breasts synchronise so you are making the amount of milk your baby needs, your breasts will naturally soften and feel less swollen. As long as your baby is feeding effectively and you respond to his hunger signals, you will usually make exactly the amount of milk your baby needs.

Tip: if your baby is only drinking breastmilk and having at least one soft yellow bowel motion, and six to eight very wet cloth or four to five heavy, wet disposable nappies a day, he is getting enough milk (what comes out must be going in!).

My baby has suddenly started feeding more frequently

Your baby may be having a growth spurt and a corresponding appetite increase, or he may be coming down with a bug and need an immune boost: the transfer of saliva from your baby's mouth to your breasts signals you to produce antibodies to any bugs your baby is exposed to and he will receive these antibodies as he drinks your milk.

Tip: take your baby to bed or relax on the couch with your favourite TV series and rest with your baby, snuggling skin to skin (this will boost your milk-making hormones) and allow him to feed whenever he shows hunger signals. This will help your body catch up with your baby's increased need to feed.

My baby only has short feeds

Although in the early days, feeds seem to take forever, often at around ten to twelve weeks, many babies seem to quite suddenly feed more quickly. As long as your baby is having wet nappies and gaining weight, she has most likely become an efficient feeder so doesn't need to suck as long. However, if your baby seems to be having short feeds and isn't gaining weight steadily, consider, is he latching and sucking well? Has he been checked for an issue such as tongue-tie (see page 280)? Is he distracted during feeds?

Tip: one indicator of a baby who is feeding well is how they are sucking. Think about how you suck from a straw: as you suck in a mouthful, your chin drops down as long as you are ingesting fluid. This is how your baby sucks at the breast and it will look as though your baby is pausing between chomps with his chin down as he sucks in milk. The longer this pause, the bigger mouthful your baby will be getting and the more milk he will be drinking. A baby who is sucking effectively (as opposed to nibbling at the breast) may finish a feed quite quickly, so be guided by your baby's sucking, rather than how long he feeds at the breast.

My baby grunts and squirms and seems frustrated when he feeds

Although some babies become impatient as they wait for the milk to start flowing, others can feel uncomfortable for various reasons. For example, your baby may be affected by tummy discomfort because as he starts sucking, this also starts peristalsis (food or wind moving around the gut) so he is struggling a bit to coordinate feeding and farting at the same time. Tired babies or babies who have been crying (crying is a *late* hunger signal), will often squirm at the breast because they are having difficulty organising feeding behaviour. This often happens in the evening, leading mums to believe they don't have enough milk.

Tip: observe your baby's feeding cues (rooting towards the breast, moving his hand to mouth and making little noises) and respond quickly. If you have been giving your baby bottles, he may be developing a preference for the fast flow from a bottle so if you do need to supplement, start at the breast then finish at the breast, so that he associates a full tummy and comfort with Mummy and breastfeeding.

My baby gulped down a full bottle of formula after a breastfeed

Sucking is an involuntary newborn reflex. Its particularly strong in babies under three months. When a baby breast-feeds, he has to work much harder to get the milk than sucking from a bottle and, unless he is actively sucking, the nipple will fall out of his mouth and milk won't be flowing into his mouth. However, when he drinks from a bottle, the person feeding the baby will be controlling the bottle and holding it in the baby's mouth so he has much less control over the flow of milk. This means that when you pop a bottle teat into your baby's mouth, it will automatically stimulate a sucking reflex. As the baby sucks, his mouth fills with milk, which he then has to swallow. The swallowing triggers the suck reflex again so your baby keeps on sucking and swallowing. It looks as though he is hungrily gulping the bottle of formula when, actually, he simply can't control his natural sucking re-flex. Of course, after drinking a bottle of formula, your baby will fall asleep for hours because he is full and also because formula takes longer to digest than breastmilk, so it's only natural that you will start to doubt your ability to produce enough breastmilk.

My baby isn't gaining enough weight

Weight gain is a useful guide and you do need to be guided by a health professional if there are concerns. However, if your baby gains weight slowly, consider if it could be a family trait. If, for instance, you are a size eight yourself, you are well below the normal percentile range for an adult woman when normal is a size fourteen, so perhaps your baby is following your growth pattern. It may help to ask your own mother and your partner's mother if they have kept their baby record books and compare these with your baby.

It is also worth considering that many infant weight charts reflect formula-fed, Caucasian babies. Formula-fed infants have a different weight-gain profile to breastfed babies and tend to be heavier after the first few months, so this needs to be taken into account when you compare your baby to the charts. The World Health Organization has created child-growth charts that reflect growth curves of infants from various genetic backgrounds and based on breastfed babies as the normal rate of growth. I have worked with mothers who have been worried that their babies are sliding down percentiles on a growth chart but when these babies' measurements have been plotted on the WHO child-growth charts, they have followed a percentile curve without any deviations.

If you are worried that your baby isn't getting enough milk and you have been feeding her according to her hunger cues, it would be wise to have a health professional such as a lactation consultant watch you feed to ensure that your baby is properly positioned and doesn't have any sucking problems that may make her a less efficient feeder.

Tongue- and lip tie

I often see unsettled, wakeful babies who have been labelled as difficult or their mothers have been urged to learn 'tired signs' – meaning cues that baby is ready to sleep – when in fact, the baby is having feeding or sleeping difficulties due to the effects of a tongue- or lip tie.

In some babies, the little membrane called the frenulum, which joins the middle of the tongue to the floor of the mouth, is too tight and 'ties' the tongue so that the baby has difficulty moving his tongue effectively. This means that the baby will be unable to bring his tongue forward far enough to latch onto the breast and draw the nipple far enough back into his mouth to feed well. If he has a lip tie – the frenulum beneath his upper lip will restrict movement so he won't be able to flange his top lip as he feeds.

Tongue- and lip ties make feeding very tiring for babies: they can't form a tight seal on either a breast or bottle so milk will often dribble from the side of the baby's mouth as he feeds, and sucking may be noisy with clicking or snapping back on the nipple as he slides off and grasps at the nipple again while feeding. These poor babies suck in air as they feed, so may be diagnosed with reflux, yet medication will not help since the primary issue – the tongue-tie – has not been addressed.

Tongue-tie is often hereditary – if either you or your partner have or had a tongue-tie (you may have had your frenulum snipped as a baby), there is a higher chance that your baby will also have this condition.

To check for tongue-tie, run your finger under your

baby's tongue; if you feel a 'speed bump' and can't slide smoothly across his mouth, a tongue-tie may be present. For a lip tie, try lifting your baby's upper lip to see and notice, does he flange his top lip outwards as he feeds or is it always curled under? If you are concerned and if breastfeeding is painful (your nipples will be pinched with each suck) or, if your nipples look squashed after feeds or have any grazes or cracks, get a professional to check.

A tongue-tie can be easily fixed by seeing a doctor or dentist who will either snip the frenulum or use a laser to revise it (the younger the baby, the easier it is). You will be able to feed your baby straight away and you may be surprised how much more easily your baby feeds – and sleeps – after this procedure.

Dummies

If you are breastfeeding according to your baby's cues to nurse, you may be told by a well-meaning onlooker that your baby is using you as a dummy. Actually, a friend who was travelling in Scotland told me of people there who called a dummy a 'dummy tit', which is exactly what a dummy is – a sucking device that imitates (albeit poorly) the real thing.

Dummies can have detrimental effects on breastfeeding. In the first six weeks in particular, babies need lots of practice coordinating their sucking, swallowing and breathing as they learn to breastfeed efficiently. Sucking from a teat – either a bottle or a dummy – requires a different sucking action than sucking at the breast so it is best not to introduce dummies or bottles in the early days if possible. If you are out somewhere and it is inconvenient to offer the breast for comfort or if you have a fast milk flow so your baby wants more sucking but would be upset by more milk, it would be better to offer a clean finger for him to suck on.

There are occasions where a dummy may be useful. It can be a lifesaver if you are walking the floor in the wee small hours with a wakeful baby and it may help soothe your baby to sleep, but do consider how and how often you use a dummy. It is best to limit dummy use to bedtime or special situations (such as when your child is feeling unwell) rather than using it as a permanent accessory.

Be aware that if you are using a dummy to space out feeds, you may be depriving your baby of nutrition. Also your baby uses his mouth to learn about the world as he explores his fingers and 'tastes' his clothing and toys. If he is sucking his fingers or thumb, you will observe that when he plays, your child will probably remove his fingers from his mouth so he won't be constantly sucking as he could be if a dummy was offered without limits. Most importantly, by plugging your baby up with a dummy, you are blocking communication: he learns to speak by practising vocalising, and if he is grizzly it is far better to listen and try and work out what is happening rather than miss learning to understand his signalling because you are using a dummy to shut him up. If you do choose to use a dummy, ask yourself, is it respectful? And what messages do I want to convey to my child?

You will need to regularly check dummies for loose or soft bits that could break off in your baby's mouth. Also understand the impact on oral development – dummies can cause malocclusion (misalignment of teeth). Orthodontic-shaped dummies are not better for your baby's mouth. In fact, you may as well use an inexpensive dummy from the nearest supermarket. Be sure to discard it by the time your baby is a toddler and certainly by two years of age in order to create the least damage to oral development.

> *Ellie had a dummy until she was two and a half. She kept it for bedtime only and when she got up she would leave it on her pillow. When I decided to get rid of it I told her a story about the dummy fairy. That night, the fairy came and took her dummy and left a little doll for her. After that she took her little doll to bed and didn't miss the dummy at all.*
>
> Melanie

Night feeds

There is so much conflicting advice about when to stop night-time breastfeeds: one book might say that when your baby weighs ten pounds he will no longer need night feeds while another advises that your baby should sleep twelve hours without a feed by twelve weeks (try telling that to a baby who hasn't read this book!). This advice is fairly extreme, but it's common to be told by a health professional that your baby doesn't need night feeds after four to six months.

In reality, many babies *do* need night feeds up to and beyond six months. From a baby's perspective, there are a number of reasons for breastfeeding at night – hunger of course is the first reason but night nursing is about so much more than food. Breastfeeding is about comfort, connection and immunity, as well as food. It is also nutrition for a baby's brain and this means that as your baby enters new developmental stages, he will most likely go on a feeding binge to fuel his growing brain. When he has been exposed to a bug, he will need to 'tank up' on the amazing immune factors in your milk and when he is in pain or uncomfortable, perhaps from teething, the relaxing chemicals in breastmilk will soothe him. Also, as your little one goes through normal stages of experiencing separation anxiety, he will want to connect to 'the source' through the security of your arms and the comfort of breastfeeding. Prolactin, that hormone that facilitates breastmilk production as well as bonding and attachment, reaches the highest levels during night-time breastfeeds. This means your baby will probably get the best milk at night.

Night-time breastmilk is rich in tryptophan, a precursor to serotonin. We now know that 80 per cent of our serotonin receptors are in the gut. Serotonin receptors affect neurotransmitters and hormones that influence various biological and neurological processes such as aggression, anxiety, appetite, cognition, learning, memory, mood, nausea and sleep. This could mean that night feeds (if an individual baby needs them; some babies choose to drop night feeds at early ages) may play an important role in development of serotonin receptors and future wellbeing.

When we consider hunger as a reason for night-time feeding, we tend to think of small babies with tiny tummies that need frequent refills to get their quota of nutrition. But older babies can be hungry too – at around five months most babies become so easily distracted from feeds during the day when there is so much to look at in the big exciting world that they get into a 'reverse cycling' feeding pattern – taking short feeds during the day and filling up during the night. Babies who are in childcare during the day can also go into reverse cycle to catch up on connection with you, to make up for the daytime separation. Babies who are developing new skills have powerful innate urges to practise rolling, crawling and pulling themselves up all day long, so their day feeds become short. It's as though they can't stop to feed because there is so much work to do. Also, think how many calories a mobile baby burns as he does endless 'push ups' or hurtles around the floor! These babies will often wake at night to satisfy hunger and to fuel their developing brains. There is no evidence that feeding your baby full of solids will be an answer either because, even if they are eating family foods, milk is still the most important source of nutrition for babies under a year old. Also, if little tummies are stressed by too much food or upset by new foods (constipation is fairly common if solids are pushed too hard), your baby could be even more wakeful and wanting to suck for comfort.

Besides baby reasons for night feeds, the most important mummy reason is maintaining your milk supply. If you have a medical condition that may make your milk supply more fragile or if you are a mother with a smaller milk storage-capacity night feeds may need to continue for many months for you to maintain your milk supply and for your baby to thrive. You don't actually have to worry about storage capacity as this isn't an indicator of how much milk you produce over all. All it means is that some mothers have more room in their milk-making glands to store a larger amount of milk. If you have a smaller milk storage capacity, and you sleep too long before emptying your breasts, your full breasts will signal your breasts to slow production sooner than if you had a larger storage capacity.

The important thing is not how much milk your baby gets at each feed, but how much he gets over twenty-four hours. This means that if you schedule your baby's feeds and space out feeds during the day, your baby will wake for feeds at night. If you have a smaller milk storage capacity, a vulnerable milk supply, a baby who is distracted or busy during the day, or a baby who has any sort of feeding issue such as low muscle tone that affects how effectively he feeds, your baby may take less milk at each feed so he will need more feeds over a day and night to get his quota. You can try offering more feeds during the day or several feeds closer together before bed to help your little one (and you!) make it longer through the night.

My second son was a big shock. He fed every two hours, day and night, and usually had a period of unsettledness during the night for at least an hour. As a tired mum I took the path of least resistance. He continued to wake during the night most nights for about an hour. I used to feed him, then he would happily play on the floor for about an hour. I would then feed him again and we would both return to sleep. I used this time at the computer to catch up on emails or write assignments.

I did a few attempts at controlled crying but found this very distressing for both myself and my son. Some days it was hard, especially when I had to get up the next day and go to work. But three years later he now sleeps in his own bed the whole night, and I sometimes miss the quiet time during the night when I could actually get some work done.

Ellen

Some mothers find a quick breastfeed is an easy way to settle a baby or toddler (whatever the reason they may be waking) and if this works for you, it isn't a problem – or anybody else's business. Night feeds have different meanings to different mothers: while many women would like nothing more than to sleep all night long undisturbed as early as possible, others cherish night feeding as a special time to share with their babies that will be remembered with fondness long after their child has grown.

One comment especially helped me cope when my babies were awake at night. Another mum said, 'When I'm up with my little ones in the early hours I feel a special connection with mothers all around the world who are awake tending to their babies.' This just struck a chord with me and made frustrating times seem easier.

There is something special about those quiet times in the middle of the night when there are no other demands (apart from those of sleep!) and you can sit quietly and enjoy feeding your baby, knowing that phone calls or visitors are unlikely . . . It's even more special when it is your second, third or more, as the time you get together is even more rare.

Querida

For now, if you are in the midst of night feeds, you can make things simpler by keeping the lights dim as you attend to your baby so that neither of you is stimulated to a fully awake state. Avoid disturbing your little one unnecessarily by changing nappies unless they are very wet or soiled. If you do change nappies during the night, it is better to change your baby halfway through the feed, then let him snuggle and relax as he finishes his feed, than to disturb him when he is all full and drowsy.

When your baby is around six months old, you can, if you like, wait a minute or two when she wakes during the night to see whether she is just stirring between sleep cycles or whether she is going to wake fully and need a cuddle or a feed. Some babies make noises as they stir but don't wake fully. By picking them up too quickly, you may inadvertently disturb a baby who would otherwise snuggle back to sleep by himself. On the other hand, waiting even a few moments may mean that some babies become more awake and difficult to resettle, so relax and do whatever works best for you and your baby.

Meanwhile, enjoy those sweet snuggles, learn how to breastfeed lying down so you get more rest, gather support so you can rest during the day if night feeds are tiring you out and remember the mummy mantra for when the going gets tough: 'This too shall pass.' It will, I promise.

All-night suckers

One disadvantage of sleeping with older babies (closer to a year old or over) is that because your baby is now adapted to your adult sleep cycle, it is quite common for babies this age to stir about every ninety minutes and, with a breast in close proximity, your baby will expect to latch on. Some babies like to sleep 'attached'.

If you find this all-night snacking disturbing your sleep, a simple trick is to turn your older baby so her back is towards you after a breastfeed (this isn't appropriate with babies under six months). This way, your baby still gets cuddles but without a breast in her face. You can break a continuous night-nursing habit by gently rocking your baby as she stirs to help her transition between sleep cycles. As she gradually drops these feeds one at a time (no more than one feed per week), she will soon be able to sleep longer. Some babies may protest a bit, but you will know best whether your baby needs to nurse for food or comfort, or if it is time to encourage him to settle without the breast.

If your baby is over a year old, sharing a bed with you and waking frequently to breastfeed, you can try moving him out of your bed onto a separate mattress on the floor (to avoid falls), making sure the surrounding space is safe. Settle him to sleep on the mattress with a cuddle and a breastfeed if this is your normal sleep routine, then move away from your baby. Often simply creating space between baby and boob will help your baby sleep longer by breaking the association between stirring from sleep and expecting a breastfeed. Also, with older babies, the movement of yourself and your partner in the bed can cause your baby to wake more often.

Of course, if this stirring to nurse doesn't bother you, it isn't a problem. Even if you accommodate your child and let him outgrow night-nursing at his own pace, he will eventually wean from night feeds whether he sleeps in your bed or not.

Night feeds and tooth decay

Fears that night-time breastfeeding will cause tooth decay are unfounded: recent research shows that breastmilk may actually impede the growth of bacteria in the baby's mouth, since lactoferrin, a protein in breastmilk kills the bacteria that causes tooth decay, known as streptococcus mutans. Also, whether you are sitting up or lying down, as you breastfeed your nipple is drawn back into your baby's mouth behind the teeth so milk is released directly into the baby's throat. This means that as milk is released, the baby is stimulated to swallow.

When a baby feeds from a bottle, milk is released

at the front of the mouth and pools around the teeth. If baby falls asleep sucking on a bottle, milk keeps on dripping into the baby's mouth, and bathing the teeth. So please hold your baby as you bottle feed rather than putting even an older baby to bed with a bottle. Apart from foods sticking around a child's mouth (clean your baby's teeth gently with a damp cloth and later, a soft toothbrush) a common cause of tooth decay is the transfer of strep mutans from parents putting their baby's dummy in their own mouths. So, if you use a dummy, never put your baby's dummy in your mouth. Instead, if it drops, rinse it under a tap or use a product such as the Philippa portable UV pacifier steriliser, which is a compact ball-shaped device, designed by a dentist, that uses ultra-violet light to sterilise dummies and teats, to avoid transfer of decay-causing bacteria from your mouth to your baby's.

Routines

One popular infant-management routine consists of variations of 'feed, play, sleep', which translates to feeding your baby, then giving her time to play and then popping her into bed. While this sounds reasonable and can help some mothers feel more in control because they have a plan, it is often interpreted very rigidly. I have, for instance, heard of babies who have fallen asleep after a feed, then been woken up (yes, really!) because they missed their playtime and the routine would have been out of whack. I have also seen mothers who have been strictly advised that they must give clear messages to their baby about what part of the routine they are following, so while the mother is 'allowed' to hold her baby while she feeds it (this is a safety issue – *never* prop your baby to feed), she must put the baby down on the floor to play and then put the baby into the cot to sleep.

> When my twins came into the world last November my husband and I desperately wanted to do everything right as new parents . . . (I was told) the babies should 'feed, play, sleep' and should go to sleep on their own in their cots. I was also told we may need to leave them to cry for a while, and that they fed far too frequently (two- and then three-hourly around the clock) and I needed to cut them back.
>
> We followed the rules and thought we were doing everything right, and that by doing so, our babies would be sleeping through the night by three or four months old. When they reached this miracle age, I was devastated to find that they were still waking every three hours through the night, and not having two or three nice long day sleeps. I beat myself up a lot – I must have done something wrong, or there was some-thing wrong with my babies! We did a bit of controlled crying, and spent many nights awake for an hour or longer listening to our two babies scream themselves silly, before finally falling into an exhausted sleep, only to wake half an hour later when I would finally feed them. We moved house when they were six months old, and their sleep was continuing to get worse and

worse, with them both waking some nights every forty minutes. Sometimes I would feed them, other times we would sit, exhausted and pat them – like we were 'supposed' to.

I was exhausted and depressed, I would cry at the drop of a hat, and was beginning to feel resentment towards my boys, so we booked into a day stay (sleep school). A week before we were due to go, my mum took me aside to tell me that she was concerned we were making it harder for ourselves. I poured my heart out and told her that if only I'd had a single baby, I would have fed it to sleep and co-slept, but with two, I felt I had no choice but to do these things that all the books told me I should. Mum gently told me that there were no 'shoulds' and that I did have a 'single' baby – two of them – and that I could follow my heart.

Something clicked in me that night, and the next day I tore up all of my parenting books and magazines (I couldn't actually tear up the books, so I sent them to the op shop!), cancelled our day stay and explained to my poor confused husband that things were going to change.

Since then things have changed. Our boys, now nearly eleven months, still wake at least three-hourly and frequently one- to two-hourly through the night. But now they are cuddled and/or breastfed back into a peaceful sleep, and at least 50 per cent of each night is spent with both of them in our bed with us . . . We're still tired, and I still long for a decent stretch of sleep, but at least now when we are woken we can simply calm our baby quickly.

Sometimes on a really bad night I wonder what we're doing wrong, and wonder if we should try controlled crying again, and then I remember that we're not doing anything wrong – we have individual babies that will sleep through the night eventually, and the fact that they need us is really a lovely thing.

Tracey

By trying to follow any style of routine very strictly, you can feel very out of control and confused when you can't make your baby sleep or feed when he isn't ready. In fact, in the early weeks, as you get used to your baby's signals that indicate he is hungry or tired or wants to spend time engaging and having a little chat to you (see The first six weeks, page 68) it may work better to follow a pattern of 'feed, play, feed, sleep'. To make this work you would feed your baby, then have a little chat and playtime and change his nappy then offer him a little top-up (you can't over-feed a breastfed baby; he will only feed if this suits him). And please don't feel stressed if he falls asleep on the breast although you may be warned against this because it will create bad habits, it can be the easiest way to settle a newborn because of the amazing hormones in your milk and the relaxing effects of sucking. In a few months, he will naturally develop the capacity to fall asleep without so much help. This way, he is likely to take a longer nap too: when you consider that a newborn will need to be fed around every two hours at first, if you have fed him, then he has had almost an hour awake, he may actually need a top-up before you put him to sleep again. Otherwise he will be awake again very soon because he is hungry.

Even if your baby seems to be 'all over the place' right now, he will soon fall into his own natural pattern and often the less you try to force this, the quicker it will happen. And, if you watch your baby and learn his cues rather than relying on the clock, you will get to know his little expressions and signals and you will develop confidence very quickly that you do know him best. You will also be able to work out a gentle rhythm to your day that takes your baby's needs into account. For instance, if your baby tends to be more settled in the morning, you may find it easier to plan outings for mornings and be home so he can have a quieter afternoon. If he takes a longer sleep in the morning, then perhaps this is a better time to be at home and get some tasks done while your baby sleeps. You could prepare dinner (make a slow cooker your best friend) to make evenings easier, especially if your baby is unsettled or wants to 'cluster feed'.

Above all, use any style of routine as a general guide rather than a set of specific instructions, and do try to filter anything you want to try with your baby by asking yourself, 'Is it safe? Is it respectful? Does it feel right?' Then do what works best for you and your baby and remember, there is a difference between a gentle rhythm and a rigid schedule.

I have come to the conclusion that I have been listening to the 'should' brigade a bit too much. Every time I'd mention that she likes to fall asleep breastfeeding, someone always says, 'You should not

*do that, it will cause problems later.' They would also
say, 'She should be on a routine!' Well, now that I
think of it, she does have a routine, her routine: feed,
play, feed, sleep.*

Astrid

Feeding to sleep

Although you may like to use other sleep cues as well as
breastfeeding, advice that letting your baby fall asleep on
the breast will create bad habits or that he will never learn
to self-settle is unrealistic and impractical: it is the most
natural thing in the world for a relaxed baby and mother
to snuggle and doze together as they breastfeed.

The soporific effect of breastfeeding is hormonally
induced: breastmilk contains a range of hormones,
including oxytocin, prolactin and cholecystokinin
(CCK). These hormones are released in both mother and
baby during breastfeeding and have a sedating effect on
both of you. Breastmilk has also been shown to supply a
type of endocannabinoid – the natural neurotransmitters
that marijuana stimulates. So when your baby falls off
your breast all drowsy and relaxed, looking as though he
is milk drunk, you could say he is actually milk stoned!

Research suggests that your night-time milk may be
even more effective at helping your baby sleep: melatonin,
a sleep-inducing hormone, is barely detectable in breastmilk during the day but peaks during the night. Recent
studies by Spanish scientists show that components

in mothers' mik can vary significantly over a twenty-four-hour period. These researchers studied samples of breastmilk taken from healthy mothers at different times of the day and found concentrations of sleep-inducing nucleotides (proteins known to have a role in exciting and relaxing the nervous system), were stronger after dark than during the day. The lead researcher of this study, Dr Christina Sanchez, advises that breastmilk should be fed fresh or if you are expressing, it is best to take note of the time you express milk then feed it to your baby at the same time of day.

With so much evidence that mama's milk actually helps babies sleep, it makes no sense at all to resist this naturally sedating and bonding process, or to wake a baby who has fallen asleep against your warm body only to try some other settling technique or plug him up with a dummy to get him to sleep again.

Please be reassured, any fears you may have that a baby who falls asleep at the breast will never learn to sleep by himself are unfounded – several of my own children nursed to sleep until they outgrew the need. One of my children wouldn't nurse to sleep and this caused me untold angst as I had to work out other ways to soothe her to sleep if we were out and she became overstimulated. What worked for us was to find a quiet space and walk with her in a carrier. At home, she preferred to be in a cradle in a quiet room.

It is true that if breastfeeding to sleep is your baby's primary sleep association, when she wakes during the night, she will expect to be soothed back to sleep with a breastfeed. If you are enjoying the closeness and convenience of nursing her to sleep, then this isn't a problem, but if it is an issue for you, once your baby is at least four months old (or older), you can gently teach her to go to sleep without the breast. Rather than resort to a cold turkey (let her 'cry it out') approach, it is kinder for your baby (and you) to make this change in baby steps. (See Sleep: one step at a time, page 248.)

Day feeds and night sleep

A study at Fukushima University in Japan which asked mothers to track their babies' sleep behaviour for six months, found that in the first few weeks babies were as likely to be awake in the dark as in daylight hours. At seven weeks, almost all the babies shifted to sleeping more at night than during the day. By twelve weeks, most (though not all) had consolidated their sleep into naps and rarely woke for long periods at night, although many still woke to feed.

If you would like to adapt your baby's day–night feeding and sleeping pattern so that he takes his longer sleep at night (and who wouldn't?), consider that each baby will need a certain amount of food in any twenty-four-hour period. It therefore makes sense that if you are stretching out daytime feeds to fit a rigid schedule this could backfire as your baby will need to wake for more feeds at night to meet his daily requirements. However, you can adjust your baby's pattern by encouraging him to take shorter spaces between his day feeds. You can try to gently wake him by unwrapping him and changing his nappy if he sleeps longer than three or four hours between feeds during the day. Then, with luck, he may take his longer sleep at night. You could also try offering a cluster of feeds closer together in the evening – many babies feed frequently in the evening anyway, as though they are tanking up for the night.

New Zealand independent midwife and lactation consultant Karen Palmer offers an interesting observation about typical breastfed babies' feeding patterns:

> I have this thought. In the wild, dawn is a time of hunting by predators and dusk is a time of grazing. Because, over the years, I have followed through hundreds of babies for four to six weeks, I notice that most behave in a similar fashion. Graze all evening, have a deep sleep, feed several times before dawn, then sleep deeply and quietly from dawn until bright daylight. I wonder how much of this is instinct programmed for protection against danger (i.e. lie still or the tiger might get you!).

Of course, flexibility is key: you can't *make* a baby feed if he isn't ready, and there will also be times when your baby has a growth spurt and will need extra feeds for a few days to match his increased appetite, which could mean more waking for a few nights too.

'Dream' feed

Another strategy you may find helpful to shift your baby's longer sleep spell to match your own is to offer a 'dream' feed just before you go to bed, regardless of when your baby was last fed. If your baby has already been asleep a couple of hours, don't wake her for this feed – don't turn on the lights and don't change her nappy unless it is absolutely necessary. Pick her up and stroke her lips with a nipple (breast or bottle). She will automatically suck and there will be no need to burp her – she will be so relaxed that she won't swallow much air anyway. If you are breastfeeding, this top-up feed should be breastmilk as formula may upset your baby's tummy or cause an allergic reaction and it will reduce the protective effects of breastfeeding.

> I cannot bring myself to wake a sleeping baby. I have tried it, with both Olivia and Charlie, for dream feeds, and both of them simply get annoyed and then fall asleep on the breast after two minutes of sucking, despite all attempts to keep them alert enough to feed. And then wake at the same time they would have woken regardless! Olivia started sleeping through for twelve hours by four months by herself, so despite me ignoring the dream feed advice, she still slept through at an early age.
>
> Lucy

While it may seem sensible to offer a dream feed rather than waiting for baby to wake after you've gone to bed, this doesn't work for everyone. Try to respect your baby's natural pattern.

By the time your baby is eating solid foods, she will probably be ready to drop the dream feed. You can either move this feed back by half an hour every three nights so this becomes your baby's last evening feed or, if you are bottle-feeding, you can reduce the amount of fluid in the bottle every third night as well, until she no longer needs the milk at this time.

Will solids help?

For optimal development, growth and health, a number of eminent advisory bodies such as WHO and NHMRC recommend that infants should be exclusively breastfed in the first six months of life. Although some health workers advise that formula-fed babies may need a more varied diet a little earlier to make up for deficits in nutrition, it is unnecessary and unwise to introduce solid foods before four to six months. Starting solids early poses a number of risks such as premature weaning and malnutrition if your baby eats too many solids and these displace milk feeds (milk will be most of your baby's diet for the first year). Or you could increase the risk of allergies by exposing your baby to potential allergens that his tiny gut isn't equipped to deal with: between four and seven months a baby's intestinal lining goes through a developmental growth spurt called closure. This means that the intestinal lining becomes more selective about what to let through. This is due to increased secretion of IgA, an antibody that acts as a protective coating in the intestines, preventing harmful allergens from passing through the gut wall. In the early months, IgA secretion is low (although breastmilk is high in IgA), allowing allergens to easily pass through the gut wall and enter the bloodstream. As these particles enter the bloodstream antibodies may be produced to them, causing an allergic reaction. These are valid reasons to see introducing solid foods as just that – an introduction rather than a meal, and to wait until your baby is developmentally ready.

Despite official recommendations to delay the intro-duction of solid foods, some parents wrongly believe that giving their baby cereal in the evening will help him sleep longer. But according to well-controlled studies, feeding solids before bedtime will not alter infant sleep patterns. Common infant-feeding advice suggests rice cereal as a first food because it is low protein and therefore low aller-genic (allergic reactions are triggered by foreign proteins). This advice started when babies were generally introduced to foods other than milk early (at around three months). At this age babies are not ready to manage anything other than runny mush but, despite recommendations to delay the introduction of family foods, this advice is still heavily promoted by baby food companies. However, in a 2011 paper 'Why White Rice Cereal for Babies Must Go', Dr Alan Greene of Stanford University School of Medicine warns of a potential connection between feeding babies refined cereals and obesity. Dr Greene advises that white rice cereal is high in calories and made of processed white flour, and likens it to feeding babies refined sugar. He also explains that first food experiences can set babies on a path of food preferences because a baby's first experiences with family foods are so exciting for parents, with lots of positive reinforcement for the baby – often with the camera capturing each messy moment. And when we mix the processed cereal with breastmilk or formula, there is an even stronger positive message for the baby, potentially creating a preference for sweet foods that can last a lifetime.

The best time to introduce solid foods is when your baby is developmentally ready and his digestive tract is mature enough to manage foods other than milk. Until about six months, your baby will still have a tongue-thrust reflex and this needs to disappear so he can transfer food from the tip of his tongue back into his mouth to swallow it. Also, by about six or seven months your baby will have good head control and be able to sit up and share family mealtimes. In fact, when your baby can sit up at the table and purposely reaches for food off your plate this is a fairly good indication that he is interested in starting to eat family foods. Another sign that your baby might be ready for food (in combination with his growing interest and developmental readiness) is that he may seem hungrier and demand more feeds but still seems hungry even after you have increased his milk feeds for a few days – rather like a growth spurt that doesn't end.

Foods that may cause wakefulness

Your baby or toddler's sleep patterns can be affected by his diet. Restlessness can be caused by allergies or food intolerance, sometimes to foods passing through your breastmilk (your baby is *never* allergic to your milk). In one study at a UK sleep clinic, 12 per cent of thirteen-month-old infants who presented with persistent night-waking for which no other causes were found were taken off all milk products when cow's milk intolerance was suspected. In most of these children, sleep normalised within five weeks, with night-time awakenings falling to nil or once per night. A subsequent milk challenge (double blind) induced the reappearance of insomnia and, after a year, when the challenge was repeated, all but one child reacted as before.

If you or your partner suffer from allergies such as eczema, asthma or hayfever, or if there is a family history of allergies, there is an increased likelihood that your baby will also suffer from allergies. The best way to protect your baby from allergies is to breastfeed exclusively for the first six months. If you are formula-feeding and suspect allergies, consult your doctor. There are hypo-allergenic formulas, but these are expensive without a script.

Food allergies in exclusively breastfed babies are caused by foods that pass into your breastmilk, not by your breastmilk itself. Allergies in infants may cause symptoms including: colic, nausea, vomiting and reflux, wheezing and respiratory congestion, dermatitis, eczema, and various rashes (although other medical causes should be ruled out for these symptoms). Because babies may be sensitised to foods in utero, it is wise to avoid binging on foods that are common allergens. A good rule is to eat a variety of foods in moderation during pregnancy and for the first year after birth if you are breastfeeding. The most common culprit is cow's milk protein (found in milk, cheese, yoghurt). Other foods that may cause allergies are peanuts, eggs, soya products, fish, wheat and citrus. However, reactions to foods seem to vary widely among individuals. Some sensitive babies react even to small amounts of certain foods in their mothers' diets, so allergy symptoms (including frequent night-waking), can be alleviated by the elimination of offending foods from the mother's diet.

Food additives are present in ever-increasing numbers in almost all processed foods and these can dramatically affect sleep patterns and behaviour. Some babies and children can also become restless after eating foods containing salicylates. These are naturally occurring chemicals which are found in otherwise healthy foods such as broccoli, grapes, apples, oranges and tomatoes as well as in some processed foods. Food intolerance expert Sue Dengate has seen remarkable changes in children's behaviour, including infant sleep patterns, with simple dietary changes, such as changing the brand of bread eaten.

I have a 10.5 month old who has never really slept. I decided to try a salicylate reduced diet. We're six days in and the change is amazing! We've gone from two

*forty-minute catnaps and waking every hour at night
to two, two-hour naps and only waking twice for a feed
over night. I'm shocked at the difference!*

Kara

Tracking down offending foods in your child's or your own diet may take some effort, especially for already exhausted parents, but in the long run it could gain you more sleep. If you think that sleeplessness may be related to foods in your diet passing through your breastmilk, keep a notepad handy and jot down your baby's crying times and what you eat to see if they are linked. If there appears to be a 'cause and effect' between foods in your diet and your baby's crying, an inexpensive and simple solution is to eliminate the suspect food for at least a week, preferably two weeks. If your baby's sleep patterns improve, you can either be thankful and avoid the suspect food, or you can reintroduce a small amount of the food into your diet – if the night-waking or allergy symptoms re-occur, you can be pretty certain you have nailed the culprit. Elimination of foods may take anywhere from a few days to several weeks to make a difference to your baby's behaviour so allergies are difficult to prove or disprove, but if it calms your baby (and you), modifying your diet is a small sacrifice.

If you are formula-feeding and suspect an allergy to dairy foods, it is not necessarily helpful to race out and buy soy milk formula, for instance, since about 40 per cent of infants who are allergic to cow's milk protein are also allergic to soy bean protein. It would be better to discuss with your GP or paediatrician whether it is appropriate to try a hypo-allergenic formula. Consult with your baby health nurse and/or your doctor before changing formula.

It can also be difficult to pinpoint food additives that are affecting your child's sleep as reactions are not necessarily immediate and may take up to forty-eight hours to present, although many parents do notice restlessness and hyperactivity after events such as eating at fast-food restaurants. After keeping a food diary, one mother tracked her toddler's subsequent misbehaviour and sleeplessness to the days at childcare when he ate pasta laden with tomato sauce. Several other parents worked out that their older babies' sudden wakefulness was related to their eating grapes.

Sometimes, sleep will be elusive without major dietary changes but in other cases it will just be a matter of balance, perhaps taking care not to overload on certain foods that seem to affect your child. A good guide to sensible eating is to include a wide variety of foods in as close to their natural state as possible. This means that eating fresh vegetables, wholegrains, fish, meats and free-range eggs, and drinking plain milk or water instead of filling your supermarket trolley with frozen chicken nuggets, snack bars, coloured yoghurts and juice boxes, could see you and your little ones all sleeping more soundly. If you find the thought of changing your diet overwhelming, seek help from an appropriate professional such as a dietician. To find out more about food additives and allergies, please see the resources section at the back of this book.

Drinking for better sleep

Soft drinks, juices and 'health' drinks often contain preservatives and almost certainly contain unnecessarily large amounts of sugar that disrupt healthy appetites and affect behaviour, including sleep. Drinks containing any stimulant such as caffeine or guarana are inappropriate for babies and toddlers – even a sip! Although some studies show that breastfeeding mothers can drink moderate amounts of coffee without affecting their babies' sleep patterns, many mothers of newborns do report restless, wakeful babies after drinking coffee, tea or cola. Newborns are particularly vulnerable to the effects of caffeine. While an adult takes about five hours to eliminate from their body the caffeine from one cup of coffee, a newborn may take up to ninety-seven hours to get rid of caffeine. This clearance time decreases with age, until at about six months it is similar to that of an adult. It can be a vicious cycle: you drink coffee (or tea or cola) to give you a hit (often after a wakeful night), baby gets a boost of stimulant through your milk and becomes more restless. If your baby is wakeful, it would be worth reducing or eliminating caffeine as the effects will be accumulative in small babies – or at least drink coffee *after* you breastfeed to give it time to clear your system.

Although they are considered to be healthy and often recommended to help babies and children sleep, herbal teas are not appropriate for infants. Chamomile, for instance, which does have relaxing properties for adults (and some breastfed babies via the milk), has been associated with severe allergic reactions if given directly to babies. Water is the safest, healthiest drink for small children and, being their most powerful role model, your own example will encourage your child to see water as the natural drink of choice. Encourage water drinking by using a filter jug and keeping cool water in the refrigerator so it tastes pleasant. There is absolutely no benefit in adding cordial – the colours and sugar may even keep your child awake. I always feel that what we feed our children is a case of 'what they don't have, they won't miss', so the longer you avoid junk foods the better. This is also a good reason to limit television viewing as little ones are bombarded with messages that they 'need' a whole range of unhealthy foods.

Booze and breastmilk

Despite worldwide research, a safe limit of alcohol consumption can't be determined during pregnancy and breastfeeding – there are potential risks to babies whose immature livers aren't able to process the alcohol transmitted through the placenta or their mother's milk. Daily consumption of alcohol by breastfeeding mothers has been shown to affect baby's sleep patterns (with babies falling asleep more quickly but waking more often), increase the risk of slow weight gain and slow gross motor development. Although many people may tell you that a glass of alcohol will increase your milk supply, there is evidence that this isn't the case. Drinking more than two standard drinks can inhibit your letdown reflex and even small doses of alcohol can alter the taste of breastmilk. Babies dislike this, so may not drain the breast. And, if your breasts aren't well drained after a feed, this can result in temporarily reducing your milk supply and it could also increase the likelihood of mastitis.

If you do choose to drink while you are breastfeeding, it is important to be aware that alcohol will pass into your milk very easily − as your blood alcohol level rises, so does the level of alcohol in your breastmilk. The good news is that as your blood alcohol level drops, so does the level of alcohol in your milk. Alcohol peaks in your blood approximately half an hour to an hour after drinking (this varies among individuals, depending on factors such as how much food was eaten in the same time period, your body weight and percentage of body fat). It takes approximately two hours for your body to break down one standard drink and your blood alcohol level to drop to zero (two standard drinks will take four hours). A reasonable rule of thumb is that if your blood alcohol level is low enough for you to drive safely, you will probably be safe to breastfeed.

If you plan to drink while you are breastfeeding, either express before drinking and feed your baby 'alcohol-free' milk or drink after a feed and wait until your blood alcohol level is safe before you breastfeed. Expressing after you drink will not reduce the alcohol level in your milk, but could actually increase the transfer of alcohol from your bloodstream to your milk. However, if you have left your baby with a sitter and you are planning to miss a feed, you will need to express enough to keep your breasts comfortable so that you don't risk blocked ducts and mastitis.

Bear in mind that alcohol will affect your responsiveness to your baby so whether you are breastfeeding or not, if you are a parent and you plan to drink, it is wise to have a designated parent (one parent stays sober and in charge of the baby) just as you would have a designated driver. Or leave your littlies with a safe carer while you party. Also, please remember safe sleeping guidelines: if either you or your partner has been drinking – even a single drink – it is unsafe to sleep with your baby.

Foods to aid sleep

Essential fatty acids are vital nutrients for infants' and toddlers' developing brains. During the later months of pregnancy and while you are breastfeeding, your baby's requirements will deplete your own stores. Low maternal levels of DHA, an omega-3 fatty acid, have been associated with postnatal depression, which begs the question, is your exhaustion due entirely to your baby's sleeplessness, or could you both be affected by dietary deficiency?

Recent research is also showing that low levels of DHA may contribute to behavioural and learning difficulties and it seems a deficiency may be linked to poor sleep patterns in infants. In a study from Connecticut, it was found that newborns of mothers with higher DHA levels showed significantly more quiet sleep and less active sleep, and less sleep–wake transition than those of mothers with lower DHA levels. In other words, they slept better. This was interpreted as indicating greater central nervous system maturity in the higher DHA group.

Fortunately, you can increase the levels of essential fatty acids in your breastmilk and aid your baby's brain development and perhaps his sleep patterns as well as your own mental health, by simply increasing these nutrients in your own diet. In a Danish study, researchers noted large fluctuations in the levels of omega-3 fatty acids in milk but consuming fish or fish oil increased the amount of DHA found in the milk. If you are pregnant, now would be a good time to address any potential deficiencies. You can take supplements of fish oil and evening primrose oil or flaxseed oil, but the richest sources of essential fatty acids are found in oily fish such as salmon, tuna or sardines.

If you are a vegetarian or not partial to fish, or have a toddler who won't eat fish, you can use flaxseed oil on salads or in smoothies (cooking will destroy the nutrients). Speaking of salads, nature's relaxant – magnesium – is found in high quantities in green leafy vegetables. Eating your greens could see magnesium pass through your milk in sufficient quantities to have a calming effect on you and your baby's sleep.

If you aren't breastfeeding, there are formulas with added essential fatty acids; however, there are varying studies on whether these have significant effects on infant brain development. Despite adding separate ingredients to formula, there are components in human milk that can't be duplicated, so whatever is added will not be working in concert with other factors such as enzymes, for instance, that may aid the utilisation of these additives. There is also some controversy as to whether adding fish products to infant formula may sensitise infants and predispose them to allergic responses in the future. Once your baby is eating solids you can offer a varied diet, introducing foods rich in essential fatty acids, or ask your health carer about supplements.

8

Baby's day

'For memory has painted this perfect day, with colours that never fade.'

Carrie Jacobs Bond, composer

For many new mothers, the early weeks can be the hardest as you struggle with fragmentation of your time and seemingly constant interruptions to meet your baby's needs. You probably feel that you would be more in control if you could implement some sort of structure into your life.

At first it is best to watch your baby and follow his lead as he sleeps and eats when his tiny body needs food or rest, but as your baby's patterns become more predictable and his cues become easier to interpret (generally by around three months), you will be able to work around these to create a gentle rhythm to your day. While predictability is more for your benefit than your baby's at this stage, as your baby reaches toddlerhood and learns to anticipate what is happening, having a predictable rhythm to his day will encourage cooperation and confidence.

A gentle rhythm

Rather than stressing about getting your baby to feed, play and sleep at specific times, it will be easier to create a rhythm to your day by taking a good look at what you need to do, what you would like to achieve and how this can work with your baby's needs and pattern.

Here's how Astrid, the mother of a ten-week-old baby, observed her baby's pattern and used this to work out a daily rhythm:

> Morning: settles quickly, has one big nap first thing, is generally happy, and enjoys playtime on the floor. Afternoon: starts to get cranky, is harder to settle, likes to be held more, but not all the time.
>
> Evening: feeds more frequently and really likes to be held. From what I can see, mornings are the best times for me to get things done around the house, afternoons are good for either an afternoon nap with the baby, or for a walk with her in a sling . . . Evenings, I think, are to be enjoyed. I would much rather sit on the couch, feed my bub (which makes her happy), watch TV, talk to hubby and have a cup of tea than stand in a dark room, jiggling the bassinette with a crying baby.

Lucy is the mother of a thirteen-week-old boy. This was her family's approach:

> We have encouraged a gentle daily rhythm since Hendrix was a couple of weeks old. I try to do the eat, play, sleep routine generally but really follow Hendy's lead as sometimes he likes to eat and have a sleep, then wake and play and we are really happy with that.
> He sleeps in his room in his cot through the night but after 7 a.m. he comes into our bed for a nap. He then has one good nap in his cot during the day, but otherwise we will be out and about and he sleeps in his pram or baby carrier . . .
> At about 5 p.m. I give him a feed then he is up for around one-and-a-half to two hours and this consists of play with me and my husband, a bath with his dad (a special ritual we really love) and a massage by me before he has another feed in his darkened room. He then goes to sleep and we generally don't hear from him then till 6 a.m. when he calls out for a feed.

Michelle, mother of a fifteen-month-old toddler, describes how she manages the days she is at home with her child:

> At 5.30 a.m. Taliver comes into our bed for a feed, then we're up at about 6 a.m. Then we have breakfast and play or read books for a little while before getting ready for work. We drop daddy off at 8.30 a.m. If I'm not working, we usually go shopping or pay bills in the morning and then come home to have morning tea and

get the washing done . . .

I usually try to give him lunch by 11.30 a.m. because I know if he hasn't slept, he will be tired by noon. Then he naps and I have some time to check my email or read a book. He usually wakes after about an hour and then we go into my bed for a breastfeed. On a good day we'll sleep for another hour or so. Then when he gets up we have a snack and I take him for a walk or we drive down to the park.

We pick Daddy up about 5 p.m. and once we get home one of us feeds Taliver his vegetables while the other one cooks dinner. Then we sit down together to eat and Taliver gets to try whatever is on the menu. After that, we pack up the toys and it's bath time with Daddy. Daddy puts on Taliver's pyjamas and reads him a story and then knocks on the wall to let me know it's time for Taliver's bedtime breastfeed. If Taliver is awake once he is finished breastfeeding, we usually cuddle and rock until he is very sleepy and then I put him in the cot and give him a few pats to settle him down for the night.

Kelly, a single mother of three, describes her day:

We have always gone with what Amelia wants but gone about our daily business too. Amelia has two older siblings (Sadie, nine, and Reuben, seven) and they have to be taken to and from school at certain times. With no family close by I have to do it all. From the day Amelia came home we did everything as normal, so if she was tired she slept wherever she was (car seat, pram, cot).

She is now very much a 'go with the flow' child.

Night-times are hectic in our house with three kids to organise and things to prepare for the next day. I try to do much of the preparation once everyone is in bed. It's too hard otherwise. Amelia has a fairly strict evening routine – to be truthful they all do. Amelia has dinner at 5.30 p.m., then her bath, then we put her pyjamas on. (She only wears all-in-ones at night, never during the day, so that she knows it's almost bedtime when we put it on.) After that we play, then we have bottle time while the other two are showering and getting ready for bed. Then, when she is getting tired, we have cuddle time and Amelia falls asleep in my arms.

By being realistic about how much you can fit into a day (some days, very little besides cuddles), there will be much less angst about how little tangible evidence you have of your constant efforts. Also, when you take away the stress of performance anxiety, things will run more smoothly and you may have better days and a baby who sleeps longer because he is experiencing a calm environment. If you despair that you seem to be achieving very little each day, one tip is to think of each thing you have done, as though somebody is taking a video of you. You will see that you do an incredible amount that isn't acknowledged. And when you find things overwhelming, take a deep slow breath (or several) to help you relax and refocus and think what you would like to experience or achieve. Instead of expecting perfection, think, How can I create little pockets of bliss? (See Look after yourself, page 283.)

We all have our own style of being: some of us find it easier to 'be' while others are happier if we 'do'; some of us are larks who are at our best early in the morning, while others are owls who have a burst of energy and a clear head late in the evening. Sometimes both parents work outside the home so timing is an issue, while others have a stay-at-home parent who can be more flexible. You may be a single parent or have a partner who travels for work, meaning you are the primary carer bearing most of the responsibility as well as the day-to-day care. It can be difficult to adapt to a child whose needs are at odds with our own rhythms but it is possible to strike a balance if you can take a step back and work out your priorities. This way, you may be able to tweak your baby's or toddler's pattern to coincide more with the whole family's needs.

Tweaking nap-times

At first your baby will pretty much sleep wherever he is – he will simply shut his eyes and doze whether you are at home or visiting, whether he is in his bed, in your arms or in the car. Within a couple of months though, a day-time sleep pattern will emerge. While some babies will happily go with the flow, it may be easier to plan around a more sensitive baby's sleep times. As one mother of a four-month-old said to me: 'My baby sleeps all night but only has one three-hour morning sleep during the day. I don't want to mess this up, so I have stopped going to yoga for now so she can have her sleep at home.' This mother sensibly worked her appointments around her baby's predictable nap-time but despite having a happy baby, the mother received criticism from her baby health nurse because, to her mind, her baby didn't have enough daytime sleeps.

You may require a different approach to make the most of daytime sleeps – again there can be some trial and error but you can work it out by observing your child and what works best for her and, therefore, what will also work for you.

> I take into account Elsbeth's activity levels during the day. If she's had an active day or has woken earlier than usual, she'll sleep earlier and possibly longer. Another thing I found that helped as Elsbeth has grown over the past year and her sleeping needs have changed (she used to sleep on and off all day and this has gradually reduced to one or two day sleeps), was letting her stay awake for longer periods between sleeps and not being too rigid on the times she goes to sleep. As she dropped a sleep, she would stay awake for longer between sleeps and if I had forced her to go to sleep at the same time as before, she wouldn't have been tired enough and would have gotten upset, which would have made it more difficult to go to sleep when she was tired enough.
>
> **Kimberley**

While some babies take long daytime naps, many are simply catnappers, especially babies who are not yet mobile. If your baby is happy when he wakes after a short sleep during the day, he has probably had enough sleep. However, if he seems grumpy and tired, it would be worth looking at what is happening around sleep times. For instance, is he waking hungry due to a rigid feeding routine? Is he overstimulated before sleep times? Creating a stimulating learning environment for babies is good, but too much of a good thing can be overwhelming for some babies and toddlers. Some babies find it difficult to move between states, for example from an active alert state to a sleep state, so they need help to wind down. It is worth doing wind-down time and incorporating bedtime rituals at all sleep times. This doesn't have to be an elaborate routine, just a simple cue or two that is transportable so that wherever you are you will be able to help your baby relax. (See Time to sleep, page 224.)

Ironically, there are some babies who will benefit from physical activity to use up excess energy so they feel tired enough to sleep. These babies may enjoy swimming, baby gym or music, or mum and baby yoga, and all babies will enjoy time spent in the fresh air, which will also help regulate their day–night sleep cycle. You don't need to organise a rigorous schedule of classes for your baby – you can do activities at home, but a baby class or two will help you see other babies in action and can help with your perspective, taking your focus off sleep as the main aim of your day. It may also give you some good ideas for playing at home, so that the end result is better sleep with less stress.

I have to respectfully disagree with 'the more they sleep, the more they sleep' advice. To the contrary, my daughter goes to sleep in record time on the days she skips her nap and is up two hours past her bedtime if we let her nap too long or too late. It is sheer hell . . . Every child is different. I don't think it helps anyone to say that all kids sleep better at night if they sleep better during the day because it just makes those of us with different sleepers feel worse.

Alex

At about two or three months old, our baby was sleeping so well at night – up to five-and-a-half hours even! But then the local nurse told me that he needed to have regular naps and not go to sleep on the breast, so I went through the rigmarole of controlled comforting. Yes, he started napping better, but his night-time sleep became very unsettled. Then I found Dr Sears' website which told me how cruel it was to let him cry and self-settle.

I was still obsessed with his napping though, so for the past four months I've been trying to get him to sleep on the breast again (which he won't). We bought a baby hammock and have been swinging him to sleep. We've been staying at home to keep to his routine, which never worked anyway, it seems. Finally, this weekend I had my brother's wedding, so Thomas didn't get his usual naps and didn't get to bed until 9.30 p.m. He was so tired that he slept all night, only getting up twice to breastfeed.

Yesterday I decided not to stress about his naps. I threw his nap routine out the window, put him down when he was quite tired and let him sleep as long as we wanted (forty-five minutes). Last night, again, he only woke twice. I don't know if this will continue but I think the answer has been staring me in the face this whole time. I kept saying to people, 'I think he seems to sleep better when he doesn't nap so well,' but I wasn't brave enough to try it as I kept reading that naps affect night-time sleep.

Bella

To resettle or not?

If your baby sleeps for forty-five minutes or so at a stint, you may be advised to resettle him. In my opinion, this can be a waste of time and energy and could simply set up a bedtime battle situation. Or you could find yourself standing over a cot patting and shushing for half an hour or longer only to get your baby to fall asleep but wake again after a quick ten-minute nap! If your baby is happy when he wakes and seems ready to play, why not enjoy his company? After some time out and about walking in the fresh air, playing in the yard or at the park, he is sure to have another, perhaps longer, sleep as he becomes tired again.

When my older two were babies, I believed the books that said 'your baby must sleep for longer than forty

minutes and you must try to resettle them'! I wasted
so much time and energy trying to get my little ones
to go back to sleep. I would spend hours patting backs
and rocking bassinettes, and even leaving them to cry.
They eventually did start to have longer naps during the
day, but I know now that they would have started to
do this of their own accord. Barclay usually naps for a
couple of hours at a time now, and he started to sleep
for longer all by himself.

Zoe

If your baby is genuinely tired (and grumpy), one way to stretch his naps is to pre-empt his waking: forty-five minutes is the length of one sleep cycle, so perhaps your little one is moving between sleep cycles and arousing but is unable to move back into the next sleep cycle. So, instead of waiting for him to wake and yell, go in and watch him when he has been asleep for half an hour and as he comes up into a lighter sleep (see Sleep cycles, page 41), put your hand on him and gently rock or pat him to help him move through this arousal into his next sleep cycle. After doing this for a few days, you may change his pattern so that he gets used to taking a longer nap.

Some sensitive babies who are easily overstimulated tend to have shorter naps as the day progresses. It's as though their little nervous systems are becoming overloaded and they are becoming more and more hyped up. For these babies it can be helpful to encourage them to have at least one longer nap during the day. Some ways to do this include wearing your baby in a wrap or carrier as he sleeps, or lying down with him and taking some much-needed rest yourself. Then, as your baby stirs, you can either rock him or, if you are breastfeeding, nurse him back to sleep. If your baby will sleep longer in a moving pram, you can either take him for a long walk or settle him in the pram and move it as he stirs to help him stay asleep – often moving the pram over a bumpy surface such as between carpet and floorboards or over a product such as the Sleep Rumbler (a rubber mat with grooves to create a bumpy effect) will help babies sleep longer. However, you do need to supervise your baby at any time he is sleeping in a pram.

Dropping naps

Each baby needs a certain amount of sleep in any twenty-four-hour period. Although individual needs vary between babies, one commonsense observation is that if your baby has more daytime sleep than he needs, he is likely to sleep fewer hours at night. There is also another equally sensible observation that suggests that good day sleeps help your baby feel more relaxed generally, so he will sleep better at night. Both arguments are reasonable but should be adapted to your individual baby.

On the first point, that too many day sleep hours will rob your baby's night sleep time, if you are worried that your baby isn't sleeping long enough at night or is resisting bedtime, consider whether he is ready to drop, or shorten, his daytime naps. Toddlers between twelve and eighteen months are generally ready to drop from two naps to a single nap each day and resisting naps or bedtime can be an indicator that they are ready for a change.

My three older children stopped having sleeps when they were about two years old (usually just as I had the next baby). But when they didn't have a sleep they'd go to bed at 7.30 p.m. which suited me perfectly. If they fell asleep in the car or such, they'd be up until 11 p.m. And even a half an hour nap would mean three hours delayed bedtime. How does that work?

Barb

You can help your child's transition from two daytime sleeps to one by extending his playtime before his first (morning) nap by about fifteen to thirty minutes each day, depending on how he responds, so that in a week or two, the morning nap time becomes a single midday nap. Keep an eye on your child's afternoon nap though, so that it isn't too long or too late in the day. If he falls asleep in the car at 4 p.m., for instance, you can expect a late evening. This is a tricky period, as is the transition to giving up day sleeps altogether, and some days your child will need a 'catch up' nap until he is ready to make the change altogether.

There is no magic answer to this unpredictable stage other than to closely observe your child and see how she manages, and to experiment with 'tweaking' accordingly. This may mean waking her if she sleeps for too long, late in the afternoon.

Busy days and sleepless nights

We live in a busy world that encourages productivity. Whether you are working outside the home or not, or whether this is your only child or you have several, it can be tempting or necessary to pack a lot of activity into your day.

Your daytime activity can impact on your child's night-time sleep. Babies and small children are like little barometers of our own feelings. If we feel stressed or spend too little time with them, they will pick up on this and demand our attention either during the day or, more than likely, at bedtime. They are also likely to have difficulty winding down and relaxing into a sound sleep and they may become wakeful at night. Some babies will even get into a reverse-cycle pattern of sleeping. This is reasonably common for babies who experience separation from their mothers during the day. Breastfed babies, in particular, may wake to feed more during the night if days are busy or they spend time in childcare.

While sleep disturbances could be an indicator that you may need to reassess your daily activities, they can also be your baby or toddler's way of stocking up on mummy-time. This is a legitimate need, not a naughty little ploy for attention (which, of course, is a legitimate need in itself).

Just as he needs food, exercise and sleep, your baby or toddler needs a quota of parent time and cuddles every day to reach optimum levels of development. One practical way of addressing this need is by doing a special activity each day, as soon as you pick up your child from care, such as having a romp in the park together. If you are breastfeeding, giving him a breastfeed when you pick him up, before you leave his carer, will help him reconnect with you – offer to pay for this extra time if you feel you are imposing or stretching the rules.

When you get home, it can be nice to take a relaxing bath together with your little one/s and reconnect before dinner and bedtime. Sorry folks, but in my view, plonking your child in front of the TV so you can cook dinner isn't an excuse, especially if you have been away from him all day, and it can create unnecessary night-waking as your child desperately tries to catch up on mummy- or daddy-time.

One way to make sure dinner is ready on time *and* you have mum and baby time, is to use a slow cooker. Put meat and vegies into your slow cooker before you leave for work in the morning, then pop on the rice steamer when you get home. While the rice is cooking, take a bath with your child, then when you are refreshed and relaxed, just add seasoning to your casserole!

Connecting immediately after work can alleviate the next problem likely to cause disturbed sleep: although it may be tempting to keep your baby up to enjoy time together in the evening, this can backfire in the form of more restless sleep as your child becomes overtired or overstimulated before bedtime. It is better to wake early and play together in the morning before work and childcare drop-off (prepare clothes and pack bags the night before). It is also worth considering co-sleeping or at least making time for cuddles in bed together in the morning, so that you and your child don't miss out on this precious connecting time.

Send a message

Just as your baby communicates his needs to you through subtle cues, you can also teach him what is coming next in his day and night by creating predictable routines and giving him simple cues that signal specific events. Even if you don't consciously introduce specific signals, your baby will soon get to know from your behaviour what to expect next. For instance, as you prepare to feed you may hold your baby in a certain way, sit in a certain chair, un-button your shirt or reach for the bottle (of milk, that is) and he will start to become excited and snuggle in, opening his mouth ready to feed because he knows what's coming.

When I teach infant massage, I show parents how to ask their baby if they would like a massage. Of course a tiny baby doesn't understand exactly what you are say-ing, but by showing the baby a specific cue each time you ask, such as rubbing some oil between your palms, he quickly gets the idea that this sign means it's time for massage. When you use cues accompanied by a simple sentence telling your baby what you are doing, it doesn't matter if things are done in a different order some days, or if you are on holiday in a different location, or you want to make a change to your patterns: as you give your baby her cue, she will respond knowingly.

You can use cues to show your baby what is happening next, to create your own special family rituals, to mark transitions in your day, and for sleep times. This way, whether you are a 'strictly clockwork' person, or a more 'go with the flow' parent, your child will feel secure and reward you with greater cooperation as he learns to anticipate events such as mealtimes, bath time, outings and bedtimes.

As you consider what rituals will be relevant to your family, look at your day. Which daily acts are consistent? Which routines do you and your child enjoy (or find a challenge)? Rituals can be little things like how your baby puts her cup in the sink or how you pop her bib on, or how she waves to Daddy in the morning. Consider how you can meet significant events in your day with meaning, for instance, with a favourite song, lighting a candle or a specific activity before or after work. If your child is already a toddler and you haven't consciously implemented family rituals, take it slowly at first – too many changes all at once can be as chaotic as no rituals at all. Waking and bedtime are significant transitions, so these are good starting points.

Screen time

Most parents don't need a research study to show them that television can affect their children's bedtime behaviour, yet in many homes the television is blaring away day and night. Often parents don't even seem to consider that this could be keeping their babies or toddlers (and themselves) awake. We don't only have television to contend with as a hindrance to infant sleep: many small children are being exposed to screens on tablets and phones at very young ages.

While all parents crave a bit of relief from the endless interaction with little ones, using technology to entertain little ones can be a short-term solution that has longer term disadvantages. One serious consideration is the exposure to radiation from phones and devices and the potential effects on children's health. Although it will take more time to draw conclusions as to the longer term effects of exposure from infancy, researchers are warning that in addition to brain tumours, hearing loss can occur due to death of auditory cells. Studies conducted by Om P Gandhi at the University of Utah demonstrated that when it comes to electromagnetic fields, children's thinner skulls and bones allow them to absorb twice the amount of radiation as adults, and because of the higher concentration of fluids and ions in a baby or child's brain, radiation can penetrate more deeply than in an adult brain.

Babies and children are very sensitive to the emotional energy around them – both on screens and your own energy as you watch a program – so scary images and loud angry voices can be disturbing (literally) and may even contribute to nightmares. There is also evidence that toddlers who aren't exposed to screens as a regular diversion become better at entertaining themselves. This natural exploration and imaginary play will set little ones up for more relaxed bedtimes too.

One American study showed that viewing television during the day or before bed adversely affected children's sleep and caused bedtime resistance, and a statement published by the American Academy of Paediatrics recommends no television viewing at all for children under two years. While this may seem idealistic or perhaps unrealistic for many parents, it is worth considering how you are using television: there are some great children's programs, but these are better watched for short periods during the day when sleep isn't on the agenda. It is also wise to get into the habit of turning the television off when you aren't watching it. This way, you won't be allowing your child to be either lulled into a stupor or hyped up by the flashing lights (they don't call it the idiot box without good reason), and you will be encouraged to interact and attend consciously to your baby or toddler. This is not only better for sound sleep but encourages brain development, learning and positive behaviour.

9

Time to sleep

*'Always kiss your children goodnight –
even if they're already asleep.'*

H Jackson Brown, Jr, author

How did you imagine your child would fall asleep – with a quick kiss goodnight and a flick of the light switch? That may happen when they're older but most babies and toddlers need help to settle and fall asleep. When I ask mothers how their babies go to sleep, I discover a range of settling techniques, and when told that a baby goes to sleep 'all by himself' it usually turns out that he has a prop that acts as a mummy substitute such as a dummy, a blanket or a lovey. This is not meant to be a judgement or criticism, but simply an observation that it is the rare baby or toddler who sleeps easily without any help. Perhaps the plethora of articles we see about bedtime battles are simply a reflection of small children expressing a genuine need for comfort which conflicts with parents' needs for convenience.

I have handed over the responsibility of putting the baby to bed to Paul . . . He is always very hands-on so the children have all been very close to him. Instead of me feeding them off to sleep in bed or on the couch, he initiates a bedtime routine (singing, stories etc.) and then lies down with them on the bed until they go to sleep. This has taken various amounts of time. I think all these techniques work better for us now because if something doesn't work (i.e. the baby isn't tired) we don't worry or wring our hands or panic like we did with the first baby but just try something different and experiment and problem-solve without the high emotion.

Maxine

Falling asleep, especially at night-time, is a major transition for little ones. If they sleep alone, they are leaving you temporarily. At various ages and developmental stages, this may be confusing to your baby or toddler, so she will cling to the security of the person she loves the most in the whole big world – you! This is why implementing a predictable bedtime rhythm can help babies and small children feel secure and will help them cooperate and relax into sleep more easily, even if it means that your presence is required.

Rather than seeing settling your baby as a negative, it can help to appreciate the benefits of sharing this precious time. Later, when your child becomes a toddler or preschooler, a bedtime routine can include stories and talks about your child's day. The trust that builds as your child confides in you is not something to be dismissed as an inconvenience to your busy life, but a foundation for your ongoing relationship with your child.

The ultimate goal is to impart the skills your child needs to fall asleep without you (most of the time) but there is no hurry and, in fact, if your baby or toddler senses your stress or urgency, this could backfire: if he goes to sleep anxious or cries himself to sleep, he is unlikely to sleep well and may wake more during the night, or he may express feelings of insecurity by becoming clingy during the day. On the other hand, a child who feels secure is likely to become more independent in the long term, so it seems a more logical choice to calm and connect with your little one at bedtime and create a positive sleep environment, than to create bedtime battles that may last beyond infancy.

Sleep associations

The term 'sleep association' often has a negative connotation, referring to the observation that whatever cue or conditions your child associates with going to sleep will be what he expects to help him return to sleep if he wakes during the night. Some people say that by allowing babies to develop an association with *any* particular cue, you are setting yourself up for sleep problems.

The theory goes that by simply placing your baby in his bed in a safe sleeping position, and leaving him to cry long enough, he will learn to self-settle without any props. As far as I am concerned, the notion of teaching your baby to self-settle and sleep all night long (because a 'good' or 'clever' baby will know how to return himself to sleep without assistance) is about as appropriate as trying to teach a three-month-old to ride a bicycle. (See The con of controlled crying, page 9.) People suggest that allowing your baby to fall asleep in your arms or at your breast, then placing your baby in his cot will frighten him when he awakes and finds himself alone. But in my experience, a baby who feels secure won't mind at all if he is gently placed into his cot after falling asleep in your presence. Most babies who fall asleep like this simply look around the room as they wake and call out with little noises that say, 'I'm awake, where are you?'

If you are feeling confused, take heart – even as adults, we all have sleep associations. Consider, how do you prepare yourself for sleep? Do you make a cup of tea? Have a bath or shower? Read a book or magazine? Do you like your bed tucked in or out, just so? And, how do you fall asleep? Do you (heaven forbid!) snuggle up to your partner as you doze off? Now, imagine falling asleep in your partner's arms only to have him or her wake you and say, 'Roll over darling, you must learn to get to sleep by yourself. How will you ever manage if I am away on a business trip?' Of course, it may feel a little odd if your partner is out of town for a few days, but most of us manage just fine and eventually your baby will too.

Bedtime routines can become cues that help even tiny babies wind down and become conditioned to fall asleep. These sleep associations can help create a positive sleeping environment, so that wherever you are you can help your baby or child relax without anxiety or battles. Over years of observation, I have noticed that children who are parented to sleep as babies and toddlers are far more likely to view sleep as a warm and comforting experience and actually enjoy bedtime. By doing the hard yards with your baby now, you are creating a positive sleep environment.

It is wise to use a variety of bedtime cues so that your baby isn't dependent on a single way to go to sleep. This way, it will be easier to change your baby's sleep cues as he grows. For instance, although a newborn may fall asleep at the breast most of the time, consider how long you are going to feel happy about nursing your baby to sleep. There is no need to stress that you are creating problems (you can gradually wean your baby from falling asleep at the breast at any age), but if this is the only way he has ever fallen asleep, it would be cruel to suddenly change the rules on him because you are over it. I would suggest that while nursing your baby to sleep is usually the easiest way to settle a baby in the early months, it is also wise to vary sleep cues. That is, don't worry if your baby falls asleep at the breast but also help him sleep by rocking sometimes, let him fall asleep in a carrier or wrap or perhaps the pram sometimes and at other times, pop him into bed drowsy but awake.

Positive bedtime cues

Here are some suggestions for a bedtime routine. Keep it fairly simple so it can be managed by a babysitter or by you when you are away from home. It also helps to carry out your baby's bedtime routine in the same order every night as they get older (so long as it is working), to convey a sense of security and predictability. Many toddlers are very pedantic about the order of their bedtime routine and will even insist on kissing their toys goodnight in a specific order. This is not a sign that your child is becoming obsessive – he will grow out of this, but for now, it can help him feel in control as his accelerating development creates changes for him every day.

Your routine may include:
- Special words or sounds
- Books or stories
- Massage
- Music
- A bath
- Wrapping
- Rocking
- Patting
- Stroking
- Meditation.

You can adapt your bedtime routine as your baby grows. For instance, a massage *and* a bath might be too stimulating for a newborn, so it may work better to give your baby a bath during the day and massage him before bed, or vice versa. And before about three months it is better to massage your baby before his bath, as smaller babies tend to cool down very quickly if they are left undressed after their bath.

> We've had the same bedtime routine for our two-year-old son almost from day one. After his bath, we all sit together as a family for settling-down time during which our son was given his last breastfeed, and now a cup of milk. Then we go into his room with dim lights, change into pyjamas and read a story, then sing 'Twinkle, Twinkle Little Star'. This has become his cue to know that it's sleep time. Then we put him in his cot/bed and give him a brief rub or massage. We've had sleep problems on and off, but we've tried to be consistent with bedtime routine throughout no matter where we are.
>
> Penny

Special words or sounds

A word, sound or phrase used each time you put your baby to bed can be a positive sleep association and is wonderfully transferable. Start using your special words whenever you put your baby into bed, whether you are also using other cues such as music or rocking or breastfeeding. Eventually you will be able to wean from some of the other cues and just use a cuddle and your special words.

Books or stories

Snuggling together for storytime is one of the nicest ways I can think of to wind down, for both parent and child. You can start reading to your baby as soon as you like – some parents even introduce a story or two while their baby is still in the womb. If you do this try a book with a good rhythm or rhyming words such as a Dr Seuss book.

Reading is an enjoyable and stimulating activity at any time of day and I would recommend that you spend many happy hours reading to your children. However, for babies and toddlers, it is good to keep a small number of specific books for bedtime only. It can be helpful to read a few stories to engage and calm your child then finish with a specific sleepy story, for instance, *Time for Bed* by Mem Fox or *The Rabbit Who Wants to Fall Asleep* by Swedish psychologist Carl-Johan Forssén Ehrlin.

We have a basic routine, day and night. I try to give TJ his daytime meals and sleeps at around about the same time of day in an effort to help his body clock sort itself out. I also have a bedtime routine that I am more strict with. It goes: nappy change and into sleeping bag, sit in rocker and give him his blankie, read Where is the Green Sheep? *(This is his bedtime book, which I only read before bed or nap-time. It usually gets him yawning even if he wasn't tired before.) Then I get comfortable and pretend to be asleep. Sometimes he cries, and sometimes he just snuggles in and plays with his blankie. At the moment I am able to put him down*

while he is still awake and leave the room but a lot of
the time I have to either put him down asleep (I usually
put him down as soon as his eyes close and he settles)
or pat his bottom in the crib until he is asleep.

Michelle

Massage

Silent nights could be at your fingertips: research from Miami University showed that infants and toddlers who were massaged daily for one month, for fifteen minutes prior to bedtime, fell asleep more easily by the end of the study. Research studies also show that loving touch has profound effects on infant development and, with just a few simple strokes, you can lull your baby into a deeper, more restful sleep.

It will only take a little time each day to help your baby become calmer and happier, with fewer stress hormones and healthier immune function. Massage releases endorphins, those feel-good hormones that help us all reduce stress and, with fewer stress hormones circulating in his tiny body, your baby will inevitably sleep more soundly. According to Dr Tiffany Field, director of the Touch Research Institute at Miami University's School of Medicine, a massage just before bedtime is more effective than rocking at helping your baby fall asleep and stay asleep.

Massage could also make your child smarter: as well as stimulating your baby's nervous system and encouraging brain development, studies have shown that babies with lower levels of cortisol (a stress hormone) in their blood do better at mental and motor ability tests. And it also helps your baby grow: in another study conducted by Dr Field, premature babies who were massaged gained 47 per cent more weight per day! Massaged babies in this study were discharged from hospital six days earlier than babies in a control group and follow-up studies showed lasting effects.

Infant massage is not only good for babies, it is good for parents too. Several studies show that mothers who suffer from postnatal depression improve when they incorporate infant massage into their daily routine, and an Australian study of infant massage and father–baby bonding found that at twelve weeks old, babies who were massaged by their fathers greeted them with more eye contact, smiling, vocalising and touch than those in the control group. Perhaps one of the most significant benefits of baby massage is that it helps you to get to know your baby and his body language and communication style as it incorporates all the important elements of parent–child bonding – skin contact, eye contact, hearing your voice and experiencing a focused response.

> I was sceptical at first that a baby this young (six weeks old) would be able to respond so positively to a massage, but it is the best thing! Claudia 'goos' and grins all through her massage – the eye contact is lovely. Her evening massage is a very special family time for our family – my husband loves it too. I think, what would I have missed if I hadn't learned massage? I don't even get that response when I bath her.
>
> **Antoinette**

When you create a special time and space for massage, your baby will soon make an association between the smells, sights and sounds around him in his special massage place and the soothing experience of being massaged. Warm the room, play soft music, and avoid harsh lighting. If you are massaging during the day, open the curtains and bathe the room in natural light. Take the phone off the hook, hang a 'Do Not Disturb' sign on the front door and have everything at hand, including nappies and a special soft blanket, towel or lambskin to lie baby on.

The good oil

Studies show that babies prefer to be massaged with oil: they show fewer stress behaviours (like grimacing and clenched fists) and lower cortisol (stress hormone) levels when oil is used. Always warm your hands first, by rubbing them together or holding them under warm water, then drying them thoroughly. Remember to clip your nails and use hand lotion regularly to soften any rough patches on your palms (yes, dads too!).

Warm the oil by rubbing it in your hands (never put it directly onto your baby) then allow it to warm or cool to your body temperature before massaging. Some babies may be sensitive to particular oils or additives, so read labels carefully to check for ingredients. A cold-pressed vegetable oil will be nourishing to the skin, feels pleasant and won't hurt baby if he sucks his hand. Don't massage your baby with mineral oils: as well being petroleum-based, mineral oils can be absorbed through baby's skin and when excreted it may take some vitamins with it. If you have any concerns about your baby's sensitivity, test a sample of oil on a small patch of skin beneath your baby's forearm overnight. If there is any reddening or a rash, don't use this oil on your baby's delicate skin. And, for safety's sake, do remember that oily babies are slippery!

Connect with your baby

Before you begin to massage your baby, ask his permission or tell him gently, 'We are going to have a massage now. I am going to pick up your tiny foot and stroke it.' Watch and wait for him to respond. By respecting your baby's attempts to communicate, you are teaching him in the gentlest possible way that he is safe: his body belongs to him, his feelings are important and he has a right to refuse unwanted touching.

Make eye contact with your baby and watch his facial expressions as you massage. Talk to him and wait for him to 'reply'. Tune in to his responses and try to understand what he is communicating to you. Feel the tension in your baby's body. Is he relaxing, or does he tense up when you touch various areas of his body? Depending on his response, you may need to stop and give your baby a cuddle or gently get him used to experiencing touch if he expresses sensitivity in certain areas. Sometimes your baby's response may mean abandoning the massage until another time.

If your baby resists massage, or if it isn't appropriate to massage her (if she has a fever, is unwell, or has been immunised within the past forty-eight hours), offer her more skin-to-skin contact in other ways: hold her against dad's bare chest, bathe with her, or hold your hand against your baby's bare back under her clothing.

Giving your baby a massage

To massage your baby, lie him or her between your legs or on your lap facing you, or kneel on the floor beside your baby. Find a position that is comfortable for you both and remember to connect with your baby before you begin to massage. It is important that you are relaxed when you massage your baby, as your stress will be transferred if you are tense. You can start massaging your baby's head or feet first, but it is important to keep baby warm, so if you undress him completely, cover body parts you aren't massaging with a bunny rug.

It will be beneficial for you, your partner and your baby to attend a series of infant massage classes, but if this isn't practical, see my Baby Massage DVD, which is also available to stream from my website. (See Useful contacts and resources, page 313.) Meanwhile, you can follow these strokes in order to give your baby a mini body massage:

- Stroke the crown of baby's head in a gentle, circular motion. Then, with both hands, stroke with flat fingers from baby's brow to his temples. With your fingertips, massage in small circles around baby's jaw. If you are massaging a young baby, avoid your baby's cheeks near his mouth or you'll trigger the rooting reflex (and he will become frustrated as he tries to turn and grasp for food!).

- Place both hands on baby's chest. With fingers flat, stroke up your baby's sternum, around the top of the chest, out to the shoulders and down to the base of the ribs and back to the bottom of your baby's sternum, making a heart shape. Then stroke gently outwards over baby's shoulders. Cup your hands around baby's shoulders, using gentle circular motions with your thumbs. 'Milk' the arms one at a time, from shoulder to fingertips and delicately massage your baby's hands and each of his fingers.

- Imagine a clock face on your baby's tummy, just below the ribcage. With the palm of your hands, one hand following the other, start at 'seven o'clock' and stroke firmly around the tummy in continuous clockwise circles (only after the cord has dropped off). This massage follows the ascending, transverse and descending colon and when alternated with bending your baby's knees up, it can be used to help relieve tummy ache by moving wind and encouraging digestion.

- Starting at the top of baby's thigh, 'milk' his legs, massage his ankles then, supporting each ankle, use your thumb to massage along the sole of his foot. Give each toe a gentle rub.

- Place baby on his tummy (with his arms forward) across your thighs. Supporting his buttocks with one hand, stroke with your other hand from his shoulders to his bottom. Finish off by lightly 'combing' his back with your fingertips, making slower and slower movements.

- As you finish a massage, it is important to gradually lighten and slow your movements then place your hands on your baby's back or stomach for a few moments: you will have created a gentle relaxed state for both of you and it may startle your baby to stop massaging suddenly. As you hold your hands on your baby, continue the mood you have created by breathing slowly with your baby and feel the connection you have made. Keep baby's clothes ready so you can make dressing an extension of the massage, or roll baby in a towel ready for a bath if this is your routine. And, of course, always enjoy a cuddle with your calm, relaxed baby after a massage!

Music

For all of eternity mothers have sung lullabies to gently lull their babies to sleep. Calming, repetitive sounds of traditional lullabies recall the womb music your baby heard before birth (your heartbeat, and fluids whooshing through the placenta). Baby music that incorporates elements such as the rhythm of the maternal heartbeat or white noise has remarkable soothing effects, especially if played continuously through the night.

When choosing music for your baby, please note that recent research is showing there are concerns about using white noise potentially causing hearing loss in babies: a recent study from researchers at The Hospital for

Sick Children in Toronto found that some infant sleep machines produce sounds that could increase risk of noise-induced hearing loss. Until researchers know more about the impact of sound machines on infant auditory development, Blake Papsin, paediatric otolaryngologist-in-chief at the hospital and one of the authors of the study, advises parents to err on the side of caution and follow the same guidelines in place for neonatal intensive care units, where sound is supposed to be 50 decibels. Papsin advises placing sound machines as far away from the crib as possible, on the lowest setting, and turning them down or off once a child has dozed off for the night.

Singing also seems to have a relaxing effect on mothers and your baby will tune into your happy feelings too. As one mother told me, 'When I sing to Reuben, if I'm distracted and just "phoning it in", he mucks around, but when I actually sing to *him*, he becomes calm and settles as he listens.' My own first baby spent time in hospital in the early weeks and later we travelled with him. I used to sing the Maori song 'Pokarekare Ana' to settle him and, despite my complete lack of singing talent, it worked wherever we went. If you are pregnant and reading this, you could choose a settling song now and familiarise your baby with the tune before he is even born, since studies show that babies remember and are soothed by music they have heard in the womb.

Bath time

The relaxing effects of a bath work at a physiological level as well as a psychological one. One of the triggers for sleep is a slight drop in core body temperature. A warm bath temporarily increases the core body temperature, then as this temperature lowers after a bath, we feel drowsy – it works for babies too. This is why timing of the bedtime bath matters. For example, it is best to have a quiet play before your child's bath, then dress her warmly and take her to bed, drowsy from the bath, for the remainder of her bedtime routine.

To give your baby a relaxation bath, rather than swish her in shallow water in a baby bath, run a warm deep bath in the adult bathtub: the water needs to be deep enough for your baby to float and should be as comfortably warm as you would have it yourself (check the temperature with your wrist before you pop your baby in). Hold your baby so she is floating on her tummy by supporting her under her shoulders and chin. If you feel a bit dubious about holding her this way, floating on her back will still help her relax. Even when she is much older, never leave her alone in the bath.

Aromatherapy products aren't recommended for babies under three months old, but for older babies and toddlers a few drops of lavender mixed with vegetable oil or milk can be added to the bathwater for extra soothing effects. Please be careful, though, about using bubble-bath products. While some baby bath products will create bubbles and only contain natural ingredients, including essential oils, read labels carefully and use all bath additives sparingly as these can cause skin and genital tract irritation that may have the very opposite effect you are aiming for – itching and sleeplessness, rather than relaxation.

Bathing with your baby can be a special relaxing and bonding time for you both or, if you and your baby prefer, you could take a shower together. One way to do this if you don't have help is to undress your baby, wrap him in a towel and place him in an infant seat next to the bath or shower while you get undressed, then take him into the bath or shower with you. Afterwards, lift your baby into his seat, wrapping the towel (placed in the seat ready) around him, get dried and dressed yourself, then dress your baby.

Wrapping

Wrapping or swaddling can become a sleep association, but this is one that will need to be changed before your baby becomes mobile and can get tangled in her wrap. To discard the wrap with an older baby, do this in steps: unwrap one arm, a few days later unwrap both arms, and so on . . . Some babies happily go from being wrapped to using a sleeping bag and, just like the wrap, a sleeping bag can signal to your little one that it is time for bed.

Sucking

Sucking on a breast or dummy has a relaxing effect on your baby and can be a helpful settling tool. However, some people say that you will have to feed your baby to resettle her during the night, or you will have to get up and replace the dummy if it falls out and wakes your baby. However, the breast really is nature's pacifier so it makes little sense to try and resist the calming effects of letting your baby nurse to sleep. (See Feeding to sleep, page 187.) If you use a dummy, you can remove it as soon as your baby has fallen asleep or while he is drowsy but awake.

It is often the sensation of a dummy slipping from the baby's mouth as he enters a deeper sleep that wakes him since his automatic reaction will be to suck harder on the dummy as it slips from his mouth. It will be easier for your baby to stay asleep if you remove the dummy as he falls asleep. To do this, as you pull the dummy out of your sleepy baby's mouth, gently close his mouth by pressing beneath his chin for a few seconds. He may make sucking motions but this gentle pressure under his chin will stop him writhing around searching for the dummy and if he arouses slightly he will quickly resettle. You can use this same technique to remove your sleepy baby from the breast.

Rocking

Rocking reminds tiny babies of the movements they experienced in the womb so it will comfort and lull most babies to sleep. This is also a sleep association that is sure to get you critical comments along the lines of: 'How do you think you will be able to rock him when he's two, or if you have another baby?' Like any other sleep association, you can wean your baby from rocking when you and he are ready, gradually and with love.

Instead of seeing rocking as a negative, it can help to understand the benefits of rocking and movement to your baby's development and why some babies seem to need more rocking than others. It seems that babies' need for movement is as intense as their need for loving touch. The calming effect of rocking your baby comes from its effect on the vestibular system, which is located in the inner ear and regulates equilibrium, making it possible for your baby to find her place in space. Before birth, as you carried your baby in your belly, she was constantly moved and rocked as you walked around, bent up and down and went about your day. So, at birth, your baby's vestibular system is programmed to expect movement. To a newborn baby with little body awareness, stillness can be disconcerting.

As you rock and carry your baby, you are not only helping her relax, you are also enhancing her development: with every movement, fluid moves in the canals of the vestibular apparatus, sending nerve impulses throughout the muscles of the body. This process helps your baby develop head and body control, which are prerequisites for learning later skills such as sitting, crawling and walking. Later, the integrity of the vestibular system is related to language development and sensory processing as well as children's ability to concentrate, to sit still and to read, so if your baby responds well to being rocked or seems to demand it, please trust that this is exactly what he needs. And, as you stop rocking your baby to sleep, consider other ways to meet his need for movement in all directions during his awake times. If you have a baby who seems to need rocking or is easily soothed to sleep by movement, consider soothing him to sleep in a baby carrier or try cuddling baby as you sit together in a rocking chair.

I used to rock him to sleep (he's now five months). I phased out the rocking by waiting until his eyes were closed, and then I would slowly stop rocking. If he woke up, I would rock again but only until his eyes closed and then I would stop again and again until he gave up and just stayed asleep. Then I would rock until he was quiet and still, then stop rocking (repeat again and again), then when his eyes were closed I would put him in the crib. If he woke up and cried I would pick him up and start over. This has been a fairly long and tiring process but it's working.

Anna

The knee jiggle, a variation on rocking, is another option which utilises movement to mesmerise tiny babies to sleep. Wrap your baby firmly and lay him on your knees, facing you with his head well supported in your hands and his feet towards you. Now, keeping your toes on the floor jiggle your knees up and down one at a time, as though you are pedalling an old-fashioned treadle sewing machine, taking care that you aren't jolting your baby. This is a useful tool if you are unable to get up and walk or simply want to remain sitting.

Patting

You can pat your baby's bottom as you hold him against your shoulder, or while you hold him on his side in his cot. If you pat while he is in his cot, when he falls asleep or becomes drowsy, gently roll him onto his back.

Although you probably won't consciously count the beat, the odds are that you will be replicating the rhythm of your heartbeat as you pat your baby's bottom. Most babies have their bottoms closest to your heart when they are heading down ready for birth, so perhaps this patting is a familiar rhythm.

Stroking

Stroking your baby or toddler's face can feel soothing and induce drowsiness. In the early days, there is a specific 'magic touch' that sends some babies into dreamland: if you stroke your little one's forehead down the bridge of his nose, you will trigger an early reflex that induces sleepiness. Although this reflex wears off at about two months, the sleep association may be set, so it is worth using this gentle stroke if it seems to be working.

Meditation

You don't have to be into mung beans or macrame to use meditation as a sleep cue for your child. It is a simple way to help your active child, from about three years old or perhaps slightly younger, to be still and drift off to sleep.

The benefits of meditation are well-documented: studies show that regular meditation can lower blood pressure and relieve anxiety and stress, so there are benefits for us, too, as we use meditation with our child.

As the mother of a very active bonus baby whose environment with teenagers in the house was very stimulating, I found meditation to be invaluable with my youngest child. At age three, while on holiday in New Zealand, he insisted on staying overnight with his older cousins whom he had just met. As they ran out the door with my baby I handed my sister-in-law our children's meditation book by Maureen Garth (see Further reading, page 319) and said, 'Try one of these to wind him down.' Her comment the next day was, 'Wow! He goes to bed easily!'

To lead your child gently to sleep through meditation, calm yourself first by breathing in and out slowly. You can get your child to do this with you by asking him to close his eyes and breathe in and out, feeling the cool air as he breathes in and the warm air as he breathes out. You can count each breath in and out if you like.

Now, begin the meditation by asking him to imagine a star in his mind. Then ask him to visualise a colour for the star, which shines down on him, 'warming' first his head and then spreading gradually down through his body to his toes as you name each body part in turn (this is called a guided relaxation).

Next, ask your child to feel his heart filling with love for people, animals or creatures (whatever seems appropriate), then his guardian angel comes and wraps protective golden wings around him and leads him to a Worry Tree where he pins all his worries. Pause a few seconds to allow your child to focus on the big tree and release any difficulties he may have had during the day, or you could gently give words to help express these. Then take your child through the gate into his magic garden, and once he is inside lead him into a story.

The length of the story and the meditation depends on your child's state of relaxation. For instance, he may walk down the garden path to the water's edge and watch or play with dolphins in the water, he may follow a bunny rabbit through the garden to his burrow where he could eat carrots for dinner with the bunny family, or he may find a circus, or fairies – whatever your little one is into. Take your time and be creative, keeping your voice slow and calm as opposed to expressive and exciting. Ideally, you will become as relaxed as your child who will drift off snug in his bed ready for sweet dreams.

10

Sleep: one step at a time

If you have read the book up to this point, hopefully you are feeling reassured that you don't have to *do anything* but love your baby and create a healthy sleep environment and he will *eventually* sleep all night long, in his own bed. On the other hand, you may be at your wit's end with exhaustion and desperately want to change your baby's sleep patterns sooner rather than later. You may be so sleep-deprived that you simply can't put the suggestions I have offered into some sort of order so they work for your baby – it probably feels as though you have a whole list of ingredients, but what you really want is a simple recipe to make your baby sleep.

While I would prefer not to be prescriptive, I do understand how vulnerable and powerless sleep deprivation can make you feel and how having a plan can help you feel more in charge. I meet many mothers who understand there are no quick fixes that work for each and every baby, but would still like help getting from sleepless nights to sound sleep. However, while there are approaches that can give immediate results (that is, a sleeping baby), these are usually short-lived because as babies enter the next milestone stage, things often go pear-shaped and this can make parents feel even more desperate and inadequate.

If you are feeling absolutely at your limit and need sleep I would suggest the following planned approach. There is no right or wrong way to go about night-time parenting, and no two families are alike. If you want to make changes to your baby's sleep patterns or where he sleeps but you can't figure out how to do this without tears (yours or your baby's), you can adapt the following approach to suit your child and your own goals. The timing can be changed, but I would caution against going too quickly or you could find yourself going backwards simply because you pushed your child one more step than she was ready for.

First I would advocate relaxing totally for a week to ten days, doing *whatever* has been working for you and your baby. At this time, it is important to take good care of yourself. (See Look after yourself, page 283.) This is also a good time to reassess your support networks. This time out will, hopefully, give you space to reflect and work out what is happening in your own life and your child's and what is most important. It will give you a baseline to work from as you begin making changes to your baby or toddler's sleep, one small step at a time. If you like, you can keep a sleep diary, but if this sounds too hard or places too much focus on how little sleep you are getting, don't add to your stress levels – this is a week to take the focus off sleep, or lack of it!

Most importantly, by giving yourself permission to ease off and do whatever works for your self-preservation for one week, you will take away guilt that you may have somehow created your child's sleep problems. If your stress levels have been rocketing because you have been trying so many different things and nothing seems to be working, your child will no doubt be feeling as confused as you are. If you are feeling pressured by your partner to let your child cry it out, it will be important to include him or her in your plan in whatever way feels appropriate. And if you are reluctantly making changes for your partner's benefit rather than your own or your baby's (apart from trying to create family harmony, which can never be underestimated), planning can be a way of easing the tension between you. At the very least it will give you time to offer your own perspective in a calm and rational way.

> Some experts suggest that children are fairly straight-
> forward in going from dependence to independence and
> that we need to assist children towards independence.
> I believe that parents only need assistance when a
> problem is affecting their ability to cope and to par-
> ent for an extended length of time. To me, children
> are like waves: sometimes they stray further out and
> their needs are less demanding, at other times (during

teething, illness and milestones mostly) they need
closeness and often constant attention from parents.
Most times, if we go with the flow of our children then
they will eventually recede again once the need has
been met. Sometimes, when we are not coping with the
needs or they have gone on for an extended time, there
are things we can do to gently assist them past the
transition period.

Melissa

The 'baby steps' plan

Starting from your baseline (what is happening for your baby) and considering your baby's readiness, work out an appropriate goal. This may be going to sleep without being rocked or fed, discarding the dummy or sleeping a longer stretch without a night feed. Working backwards from your goal, break your task into baby steps so you can change just one thing at a time.

As you take each tiny step in the direction of your goal, be prepared to stick with every change for seven to ten days to give it a chance to work as your baby adapts (unless your baby is upset, then you would go back to base and try again in a few weeks). For instance, you may want to help your baby learn to settle in his cot without breastfeeding to sleep. Remember, it is unfair on your baby to change the rules that you have created by making him go 'cold turkey'. Perhaps substitute a cue that is more easily discarded at this transition time. For example, playing music. Remember, too, that this is an unrealistic expectation for a baby less than four months old.

Week one: Add gentle lullaby music to your baby's bedtime routine as you breastfeed her to sleep. Play this music on a low volume at every sleep time – the idea is to get your baby used to the music so it has a relaxing effect and she begins to associate it with bedtime. You can't expect that any music, whatever promises are written on the packaging, will have magical effects on your child's sleep if you haven't used bedtime music before now. Simply substituting music for whatever sleep cues your baby is accustomed to is more likely to create a stress response than the desired aim – a relaxation response. So experiment with music at quiet times during the day. What seems to help her relax?

Week two: Keep playing the music, which he will now associate with sleep, and take him off the breast (or remove the dummy, if this is your goal) while he is drowsy but awake. As you remove the dummy or breast, gently close your baby's mouth and press beneath his chin for a few moments to discourage him from re-latching. Rock him a little and hum or say your sleepy words if you have introduced these and let him fall asleep in your arms but not on the breast (unless he is upset, then offer the breast until he settles and relaxes, then try again).

Week three: Breastfeed your baby as you play his sleepy music, then place him into the cot while he is drowsy but awake. Keep your hand on him and place your face next to him, maintaining eye contact. You can hum or say your sleepy words if this seems to soothe your baby. You can rock him gently in the cot on his side facing you and lay him on his back when he falls asleep. Alternatively, you can hold your baby on his side with one hand and gently pat his bottom with the other hand.

Week four (or when baby is consistently settling in the cot): Play the music, but gradually withdraw contact. Rock less as you place him in the cot, just place your hand on him comfortably and say your goodnight words.

When your baby has gone down happily for at least five days, you can either breastfeed him ten to fifteen minutes earlier, put him in his cot awake as you say his sleepy words and let him fall asleep to the music only, or get your partner to put him to bed (this is especially helpful for older babies). This helps gently wean your baby from the association of breastfeeding to sleep. If he cries, pick him up, cuddle him until he is drowsy, then pop him down again. If cuddling doesn't settle him, offer the breast and move back a step until he is happy to settle with an earlier breastfeed, then a bedtime cuddle and being put in his cot drowsy but awake listening to his music.

Just make this change at bedtime and do what you normally do to comfort and resettle when baby wakes during the night. You don't need anxiety around night-time awakenings and in any case, within a couple of weeks of being able to settle himself to sleep at bedtime, your baby may sleep longer without any intervention or extra angst for either of you. If your older baby doesn't resettle during the night within a couple of weeks, try extending him by using the baby-steps process for one night-waking at a time, rather like a weaning process. It is also best to work on changing the night-time routine at first before making changes to nap-time cues.

Eventually, you can wean your baby off his sleepy music by reducing the volume of the music several weeks or months later, but really, a bit of gentle music is hardly an inconvenience. Some parents find that playing the sleep music continuously on a low volume overnight helps cue baby to fall back to sleep during the night. Remember though, not to place music too close to your baby and keep it on a low volume so you don't risk any harm to his developing sense of hearing.

The key to lasting change is to take baby steps. If you have an older baby (nine to eighteen) months, you may be able to move through the steps a bit faster – some parents have made changes over several days but please let your baby be your guide. If you are trying to wean an older baby or toddler from bedtime breastfeeds, after you have got him used to other bedtime cues, try getting your partner to settle your little one – the sucking-to-sleep association can sometimes be changed quite quickly if Dad is doing the settling. Again though, if your baby is very distressed, please take a step back – there is a difference between breaking a habit and ignoring a need and your baby will be your best guide to which one you are dealing with.

Night-time weaning

It is not uncommon for older babies to wake repeatedly during the night for a bottle or breastfeed through the first year and beyond. (See Night feeds, page 174.) It isn't fair on your baby to wean cold turkey and if you are breastfeeding and wean too quickly, you are likely to suffer from painful engorgement.

You can attempt this by progressing in baby steps from the bedtime changes (as above): if your baby has been going to sleep happily without a bedtime bottle or breast for at least two weeks, you may want to move to the next step, stretching the time between feeds and dropping one feed at a time, losing no more than one feed a week. This is a slow and steady process but it has more long-lasting results as it accommodates your baby's needs and can be tailored to his individual readiness. Each layer of this approach will set a foundation for the next stage of change: for instance, once your baby has learned to settle to sleep without a breastfeed or bottle at bedtime, he will find it much easier to settle during the night with a quick cuddle or pat and his sleepy words. If he protests, then he probably isn't ready yet or he may be expressing a need for reassurance, physical contact or a drink (try offering water or let Dad offer water and a cuddle).

If your toddler wakes for bottles of milk overnight, one way to wean is to gradually reduce the amount of milk in the bottle and/or water the milk down over a period of a few days or a couple of weeks – whatever works with your child. A caution though, please don't water down any bottles of formula or expressed breastmilk for a baby under a year. Milk is the most important food for nutrition under a year and if you have a baby younger than six months any water can dilute the sodium in the baby's bloodstream to the point where 'oral water intoxication' develops, and this can lead to symptoms like low body temperature, bloating, and seizures.

For an older toddler who is able to talk, night-weaning could be a matter of gentle negotiation. Before you spring it on your toddler that the milk bar is closing overnight, it's much kinder to start the process by helping him understand the difference between day and night. Most little ones can grasp this concept by around eighteen months but often it can take longer for toddlers to manage night-weaning without becoming upset, especially if they are currently getting molars, are separated from you during the day or are going through a major developmental leap. Start by talking about day and night: greet the day and say goodnight to the moon, read simple stories about night-time and sleeping. Then introduce the concept of having 'boobie' when the sun shines – there is a beautiful children's picture book *Nursies When the Sun Shines* by Katherine Havener and Sara Burrier that helps to sow the seeds of cuddling at night but waiting until morning to breastfeed.

There is no age that you should night-wean – if it's not a problem to you, it's not a problem – and even if you don't actively initiate weaning, your little ones will drop night feeds of their own accord as they start sleeping through. Your milk supply will reduce accordingly and night feeds won't be so attractive, so you will easily be able to offer a sip of water if your little one seems thirsty. Trust your baby and your own intuition – you will know what feels right for her, how you are managing and when it is time to make changes.

My babies have all fed through the night till about eighteen months or so. They also (or at least the first two) had periods of sleeping through, sometimes for months at a time . . . With Angus, my last one (he was two yesterday), I was becoming frustrated in the last few months as he was still feeding four or five times in six or seven hours. So about two months ago I put my foot down.

The girls only ever fed a few times a night (regularly three times or less). With all of them I actively night-weaned them when I felt I'd had enough . . . This was very subjective on my part. Paul was not part of the decision-making. I only know that it was a gut feeling that they could cope with me saying no. Paul would take over the night care and I retired to another bed-room. Paul offered them comfort and a drink of water but no milk. We also explained to them that there was no more milk until the sun came up.

The two girls were about eighteen months and after two nights they slept through without asking. Angus was much more reluctant and this technique did not work for him. I ended up night-weaning him while Paul was away overseas for two weeks and just said no and made lots of 'shushing' noises. He was comforted as long as he could hold on to me.

Once the night-weaning was well established we moved the second and third children in with the sibling next up in the line. They have a queen-size bed and sleep together. Ella, who is now ten, begged at Christmas last year for her own bed and bedroom. We set her up only to find the novelty has worn off and her sister's loneliness got the better of her and so she is mostly back in with Lucy who is six. Angus has now joined them since he has given up the night-feeding, but he often joins us in our bed during the night. Lucy hardly ever came back to our bed once she left it and slept the whole night through consistently until Ella moved out.

Maxine

I tried night weaning when Poppy was about sixteen months but she was very upset, so I waited until her molars and canines were through and at around twenty months I started with her first night wake-up and told her my boobs were empty. She was grumpy but not really upset and went back to sleep with a cuddle. After a few nights of refusing the first night feed, I told her I was empty for her second wake-up. After a few nights she was happy to have a cuddle when she woke at night. No tears, and she now sleeps through until early in the morning, just having a breastfeed at bedtime and in the morning – she is almost completely weaned.

Melissa

Waking an older baby

You are probably thinking, what is going on here? She must be crazy to think I would wake a sleeping baby, especially when all I want is sleep! Actually, if you have a child over twelve months who is otherwise happy and feeding well but wakes at exactly the same time each night and needs a bottle or breast, this approach, which is the reverse of controlled crying, can work surprisingly well. It does require you to be very organised and will mean some extra wakefulness for you for a few nights, but the benefits include more uninterrupted sleep. Think of it as short-term pain for long-term gain!

First, start by reducing the amount of milk you are giving your baby when she wakes at night, so she will get used to taking this nourishment at other feed times. Otherwise, it would be rather like expecting us to suddenly stop eating breakfast or dinner or at least cutting out morning tea. You can either breastfeed for a few minutes less or gradually reduce or water down the amount of milk in your baby's bottle until she is having a very small feed. Sometimes this will be sufficient intervention to stop the waking but if it isn't, the next step involves the waking process.

The theory goes that if you pre-empt your child's wake-up call, and wake *him* instead, you will reset his sleep cycle and break his regular pattern. In practice, set your alarm for half an hour before your baby would normally wake, then gently wake him, be pleasant and cheerful (but not noisy), give him a cuddle and tuck him back to sleep. Each night, progressively wake him another fifteen minutes later so that you gradually move his waking time forward. Soon he will be sleeping longer and will, hopefully, stop waking habitually at this time.

Regaining trust

It is not uncommon for babies who have experienced sleep training, separation or trauma (such as a hospital admission), to exhibit fear and resistance about sleep or about their cots. If you have tried controlled crying or have been separated from your child, and now your baby is refusing to go into his cot without screaming the house down, or he is hyper-vigilant and clingy, or more wakeful then ever, don't despair. You can regain your baby's trust.

The first step in helping your baby overcome her fears about sleep is to work on your relationship with her throughout the day, not just around sleep times. It is better to give up all notions of teaching her to sleep at this point, because you are going to have to work through her anxiety around sleep and separation issues before you can make any changes.

Think of the elements of bonding – touch, eye contact, the sound of your voice, the smell of your body and your responsiveness to his communication. Depending on the age of your baby or toddler and his activity level, you could try reconnecting through massage. Don't expect him to start off naked and let you give him a full massage – if he's mobile he probably won't stay still long enough anyway. Instead, try to create some special time when your little one is calm and sitting on your lap or next to you and start by stroking his legs or rubbing his back beneath his shirt. Gradually increase this touch as he feels comfortable. Another suggestion is to take baths or showers together.

The ultimate trust builder after any trauma is co-sleeping, whether your child is in your bed or you move his bed next to yours or sleep together on a mattress or futon so that there is no risk of him falling off the bed if you are not in the room. Create a nest and settle your child with cuddles, staying with him as he falls asleep. At first, you will need to stay with him while he sleeps too. Remember, your presence is the quickest way to teach your baby he is safe at sleep times. Get a good book to read, catch up on some paperwork or have a rest. Think of this as an investment in your own wellbeing as well as your child's. At this time you can introduce one or two gentle sleepy time rituals – perhaps a story or music.

Be prepared to hold your child as he falls asleep and don't even attempt to pop him into the cot. At first, for daytime naps, you might take a walk and let your child fall asleep in a carrier or in his stroller. A distracting activity that tires him such as a swim, a play in the park or perhaps a mum and baby exercise class will help him feel tired and connected to you, so he is less likely to resist sleep. Once your child stops fighting sleep, you can move to the next step – helping him feel safe in his cot again.

Soon, you can reintroduce the cot by popping some safe toys into the cot and encouraging playtime or story-time while you sit nearby with your child (with the side down) but only for short spells at first. Gradually increase playtimes in the cot as your little one seems happy. If you haven't already done so, move the cot into your room and even against your bed. Later, you can gradually move the cot further away – from beside your bed, to the end of your room, and when the timing seems right, into your child's own room.

Meanwhile, keep up the connecting cuddles, massages and bathing together and, as trust is restored, you can try daytime sleeps in the cot – at first cuddling your baby until he is very sleepy, or even asleep before you place him in the cot. Remember to take it very slowly. This may all seem terribly inconvenient, but if sleep training or some other traumatic experience has resulted in a clingy, stressed child it will take time to heal this anxiety. However, it will be worth the effort as your baby becomes confident again and your connection with him is restored. Your child's sense of trust is a cornerstone of his mental health.

From cot to bed

When your child can climb out of his cot, he is ready for a bigger bed. The specific age varies as much as infant temperaments: one child will seem to have monkey glands and be swinging a leg over his cot sides even before his first birthday, while another might placidly play until you come to get him, until he is three years old.

Also consider the amount of room your child has in a cot. If your older baby or toddler is big or a restless sleeper, he may sleep more soundly on a futon or mattress on the floor where he will not be woken by bumping himself on the cot sides. Some parents use a mattress on the floor as a transition space from cot to bed. Others transfer their child from a cot directly to a single bed. To maintain a safe sleeping environment you will need to do a safety check of the room through the eyes (and climbing ability) of a mobile toddler. If he is an early morning waker (and wanderer) shut doors to rooms that are potentially unsafe such as toilets and bathrooms and take care not to leave low windows open that he could climb through and perhaps put a door gate on his room so he will have to call out when he is awake and ready to explore.

Generally, by the age of two or older, it is fairly easy to move your child out of a cot into a bigger bed. There are a few provisos though: if your child is experiencing other changes such as starting childcare, toilet training, weaning or you have a new baby, it would be sensible to wait until she adapts to these changes before you also alter her sleep arrangements. If you are expecting a new baby it is best to make changes well ahead of time if you want to put the new baby into your toddler's cot. A good rule of thumb is to avoid major changes from three months before to three months after you have a new baby.

The best way to enlist your child's cooperation as you change his sleeping space is to involve him in the process. Take him to choose a new doona and his own pillow.

You can break this big change into baby steps if you like, by popping your toddler to sleep in her big bed during a daytime nap at first, then progressing to night sleeps. If you are moving her into a new bedroom, it is a good idea to let her play in there and gradually move her toys into her room several days or weeks before the move, as you prepare her own room. Talk to your little one about the move – be matter-of-fact and positive. If she senses it's a big deal to you, it might become one to her and create unnecessary resistance.

If you have a bedtime routine, continuing this will help with the transition from cot to bed, but you may have to stay with your little one until he is drowsy or even asleep before you leave the room, or you could find yourself taking him back to bed over and over. If you keep bedtime calm, staying with your child shouldn't take too long or be a burden: if little ones have happy associations with bedtime, they will see bed as a comforting place when they are tired and stay there without a fuss – and this is where all your earlier responsiveness to your baby will pay off.

> At night-time I would tuck them into their bed, then lie down next to them with a book and book light. That way they fell asleep with security, and also couldn't get up and play! I did this with the older two. With my youngest (who is now four), I had a different tack. We put a cot mattress on the floor next to our bed and I would tuck him up and say good night, then leave. He would promptly get up and play for a bit and then go and lie down and sleep. Eventually he moved into the shared room with his siblings.
>
> **Louisa**

11

Evening pains

*'Over my slumber your loving watch
keep – rock me to sleep, mother,
rock me to sleep.'*

Elizabeth Akers Allen

Little ones seem to be much more bothered by discomfort or pain at night-time and it also seems common for children to present with symptoms of illness during the night. This could be due to the fact that during the day there is more stimulation to distract them from their discomfort or that some pains such as sore gums or earaches are made worse by lying horizontal. One of the most frustrating aspects about being up all night with a sick child is that often by morning, your little one seems to have made a remarkable recovery and you probably feel like a fraud taking her to a doctor. A good rule of thumb here is that if you couldn't stand another night like the one you have just suffered, it would be good insurance to have your child checked.

There are some conditions that come under the category of sleep disorders such as sleep apnoea, or perhaps your child's disturbed sleep is due to enlarged adenoids or tonsils. If your child snores or you have concerns that a health issue may be affecting her sleep, do check with your doctor. In fact, any time you are worried about your child's health seek a professional opinion. Don't ever worry that a doctor will dismiss you as an overanxious parent (if so, find a new doctor) or that you may be wasting their time – you are paying for peace of mind.

If your child has woken at night with an illness such as croup or asthma or has required a hospital trip, he may have some fears about sleeping for a while afterwards. It is important to be patient and supportive as he overcomes these, without reminding him of his frightening experience.

Finding a doctor

There is a range of care options for your unwell children from a local general practitioner (who knows you and your child and will have your family's records at his fingertips) to a large medical clinic (which will usually be open longer hours) or a hospital. As a parent, it is wise to know where all these facilities are and which is your nearest hospital casualty department. If your nearest casualty department is part of a private hospital, do you have to pay on attendance, or can you take the bill with you to be paid later? Are you eligible for a Medicare rebate, or can you claim the costs on private health insurance?

If you don't already have a family doctor, there are a few things to consider when you go doctor shopping. Think about what your priorities are in relation to what is offered at local medical clinics. Some general practitioners have extra qualifications in paediatrics; some clinics specialise in women's and children's health; some doctors have a better rapport with parents and children and may be much more empathetic and helpful towards families with sleep issues. It is also worth considering the availability of your doctor – can you get an appointment easily and how long are you likely to sit in a waiting room with a cranky baby before you are seen? Ask other parents about their doctors and why they have chosen that particular person.

Help your doctor

To describe your baby's symptoms accurately, it can help to write notes before you make your phone call to the clinic or emergency department: it's very difficult to maintain a clear frame of mind on barely any sleep and you may need to convince a receptionist that your baby really is unwell and that you do need an appointment today!

Here are some questions your doctor may ask you:
- What is your baby's temperature?
- How long has he had a fever?
- Is your baby lethargic? Cranky? Whimpering?
- When did he last feed?

- How much is he drinking?
- Has he tried any new foods recently?
- Does he have a rash?
- Is his skin pale, flushed or mottled?
- What colour is your baby's urine?
- Is your baby pulling at his ear? Is his ear red?
- Has he been vomiting? How many times has he vomited? Is there any blood in his vomit?
- When was his last bowel movement? What colour was it? Was it hard, runny or frothy and did it contain mucus or blood?

Ask your pharmacist

Whether you buy an over-the-counter remedy for your baby, or whether you have a doctor's prescription for medication, asking the pharmacist a few questions (*before* you leave the pharmacy) can prevent confusion when you have a screaming baby and a dose of medicine vomited down your shirt. In your fragile (read, confused and exhausted) state (the normal state for parents of crying babies), these questions can also act as a checking system for you – that you have picked up the correct prescription and you do understand the dosage instructions.

- What is the name of my child's medicine?
- What symptoms will it relieve?
- What is the dosage?
- How is the medicine administered?
- Can it be taken with other medications?

- Is it best given before or after food?
- Do I have to wake my baby to give medicine during the night?
- How long will my child need to take this medication?
- Are there any side effects?
- What should I do if my baby experiences side effects?
- What should I do if my baby refuses or vomits the medicine?
- How should the drug be stored?

Alternative practitioners

Some parents report improvements in their baby's sleep patterns after treatment with complementary therapies such as naturopathy, aromatherapy (this is not appropriate for babies under three months old) or homeopathy. Others find relief after treatments by alternative practitioners such as a paediatric chiropractor or a cranial osteopath. When you seek help from any health carer, it is wise to check thoroughly whether they are qualified and experienced in treating infants and children and whether they belong to a recognised professional body.

Sleep and pain

Although they don't constitute a medical emergency, there are some conditions that are associated with poor sleep patterns and night-waking in infants. It is useful to be aware of these and how you can support your baby if his waking is associated with discomfort from the pain of teething, colic or reflux.

Teething

Some babies are barely bothered by teeth erupting, while others (even if they are normally the most placid beings) will turn into little aliens who cry, develop sleep problems and want to breastfeed frequently for comfort. To help your older baby or toddler sleep more comfortably when he is teething, try elevating the head of his cot a little: this will relieve some pressure and will also reduce the chance of gagging on saliva, as your baby will have more drool while he is teething. It is best to try this during the day at first so you can see how your baby responds and that he is sleeping safely.

Some teething babies may refuse to feed or bite down hard with their sensitive gums (biting seems to relieve sore gums). If she bites the breast that feeds her, don't get angry – she doesn't realise she is hurting you – but there are things you can do to prevent or stop your baby biting during feeds. Babies can't actively feed and bite at the same time so generally when your baby starts to bite it is usually towards the end of a feed. By watching your baby closely as he breastfeeds, you will get to know the cues that tell you he is almost finished feeding and/or likely to bite – some babies will start to fidget, pull off the breast and look around, or even tense their jaws right before they clamp down. Keep your finger ready to pop between baby's jaws and remove him from the breast before he starts to bite. This may mean that your baby gets fewer comfort feeds for a while, which is a pity as a teething baby is easily comforted at the breast. However, in the long run it could mean that the breastfeeding relationship will continue longer. After all, even the most devoted mother won't want to keep breastfeeding a persistent biter.

If your baby seems to be biting as he ends a feed and gets tired or starts slipping off the nipple, instead of disengaging him, it can often be more effective (and less painful to you) to try pushing him closer to the breast. As his nose pushes against the breast he will need to open his mouth wider to breath so will reposition himself at the breast and re-latch correctly.

If your baby bites at the start of a feed you may find offering cool food to chomp *before* breastfeeding helps relieve sore gums and baby then feeds nicely. Try offering your baby alternatives (to your breast) to gnaw on – a clean, wet face washer that has been in the freezer or a cool teething ring. If she is eating solids, a frozen bagel or frozen slices of banana or cool watermelon can feel good to swollen gums.

Some babies bite when they become distracted or they take a nipple with them between their teeth as they turn their heads to look around. Try breastfeeding in a quiet space and give your baby your full attention as she nurses – make eye contact, stroke your baby and encourage her to be gentle by talking quietly and telling her, 'Good girl, gentle, gentle'. Many mums have found another great way to help older babies stay focused on breastfeeding, especially when out and about where it is difficult to find a quiet space, is to wear colourful baby-safe beads. Babies are engaged by the bright focus beads and tend to touch and play with these during feeds instead of pulling off and on the breast to look around.

Yelping in shock when baby bites may frighten a sensitive baby and could encourage breast refusal or it could simply make your baby laugh and try biting even more to elicit such a hilarious reaction. Instead of reacting (easier said than done!) it is better to carefully slide your finger into baby's mouth between her jaws and remove her from the breast. You can gently but firmly tell her, 'Don't hurt, Mummy.' Then distract her. If you feel she may still be hungry try feeding again in a few minutes. If an older baby bites and laughs at you or your baby is a persistent biter, it is reasonable to remove him from the breast and pop him on the floor for a few minutes – this will soon give him the message that biting means the feed is over.

If your teething baby won't feed, you could try nursing when she has fallen asleep – pick her up gently without waking her and hold her to the breast. If you are concerned about your baby's fluid intake, sucking on homemade icy poles made from expressed breastmilk, formula or diluted fruit juice may be comforting. Ask your doctor about teething remedies.

To help ease painful gums:

- Rub baby's gums with your finger (wash your hands thoroughly first).
- Chill a teething ring in the freezer (don't ever hang teething rings or dummies around your baby's neck

as the cords pose a strangulation risk).

- Let him chew on a wet washcloth or a frozen piece of apple inside a muslin cloth (to prevent choking on chewed-off pieces of apple).
- If baby has started eating solid foods he may enjoy chilled soft foods: a frozen slice of banana or a frozen half banana with an icy-pole stick poked into it will 'mush' down as baby gnaws on it (with supervision, of course) or try ice-cold apple puree. Never give hard foods such as carrot, which may be a choking hazard.

Colic

Colic spells are most likely to be worst in the evening when mothers' and babies' reserves are lowest. Although you may feel inadequate and blame yourself for your baby's colic, especially if you are a first-time parent, take heart – neither your inexperience nor your nervousness is causing your child's pain. Your tension is a perfectly normal response to your infant's distress, not the cause of it.

The term 'colic' is derived from a Greek word, *kolikos*, and is used to describe an acute, sharp pain in the abdomen. This pain was once thought to be caused by gas in the stomach, so mothers diligently burped babies after feeds to bring up swallowed air in order to prevent colic. The theory goes that swallowed air would later cause pain as it became trapped in the intestine. These days, infant colic is attributed to other causes.

Neonatal paediatrician Dr Howard Chilton explains that although the baby looks as though he is in excruciating pain, colic is not about pain but rather, overstimulation of the baby's immature nervous system. In an interview, he described this to me as a 'pain in the brain' and recommended reducing stimuli and helping the baby to 'reset' his nervous system by retreating to a quiet, dimly lit or darkened room with your baby for up to twenty-four hours.

It seems that 'colicky' babies may be less able to tune out stimulation or move smoothly from one state of consciousness (such as sleeping or being alert) to another, remaining stuck in this crying state. However, as the nervous system matures at about three to six months, the baby, thankfully, calms down.

Meanwhile, there are things that may ease your baby's crying and help her get some rest: firstly, responding to your baby's cries promptly has been shown to have a more calming effect and will reduce crying in the longer term. According to Dr Chilton, you can reset your baby's overstimulated nervous system by 'boring your baby'. In other words, reduce the stimulation to your baby by snuggling together in a darkened room, holding your baby against your bare chest where she can hear your heartbeat. Breastfeed, snuggle and stay in your bedroom for at least a day, preferably two days – away from visitors handling and passing the baby around, noise from television and other children (if this is possible – we don't all have helpers available).

Swaddle your baby or wear her against your body and when she is asleep or drowsy you can try popping her down in her cot. Some babies will respond to rhythmic patting, others will find this too stimulating so will be better just being gently rocked with one hand on them to help them settle if they arouse as you transition them into the cot.

Whatever the causes of your baby's colic, or whatever time of day your baby typically cries, coping strategies could include being prepared for your little one to need extra care during his witching hour. If your baby has an evening fussy time, for instance, try to complete other tasks during the day: make dinner in the morning, or cook double quantities and keep some extra meals handy in the freezer. If your baby usually cries late in the evening, you might feel more prepared if you have everything at hand (including your car keys and relaxing music in the CD player) so you can give your baby a relaxation bath, feed or ride around the block – whatever works best. You might feel more relaxed if you have your own bath or shower and some together time with your partner or a quiet cuppa before baby starts crying. Plan quiet evenings and try to snuggle up and have a nap with your baby during the late afternoon. Pre-empt (and possibly prevent) your baby's crying time by giving him a massage or a relaxation bath half an hour or so before his anticipated witching hour.

Although massage is not a simple quick fix and is best introduced when baby is calm, massage can release relaxing hormones in you and your baby as you massage so it will help reduce a stress response in both of you, creating a calmer environment and helping soothe the sobs (yours and your baby's). Abdominal massage should not be used until your baby's cord has dropped off or if your baby is crying in obvious pain. Take your cues from your baby: if he is distressed, it may be more helpful to simply snuggle him against your bare skin. For simple massage techniques, see my Baby Massage DVD – this can be accessed as a streaming video from my site pinkysbabymassage.com.

Reflux

Your baby is irritable, grizzly, hates lying on his back, spits up or vomits often, has hiccups constantly and he is a nightmare to feed: he starts to feed voraciously, then he wriggles, squirms and throws himself off the breast or when he isn't doing this, he wants to be permanently attached to your breast. He screams after and between feeds – waking from a deep sleep suddenly screaming as though somebody has poked him with a pin!

Take heart – it's not your fault. Your baby is unhappy because he is uncomfortable or in pain. The symptoms just listed can be a red flag that your baby may be suffering from gastroesophageal reflux, or reflux, as it's commonly called.

At first, all babies will have reflux to some degree, because their digestive systems are immature. At the bottom of the oesophagus there is a ring of muscle that helps keep contents in the stomach. In babies, this sphincter cannot squeeze shut as effectively as it can in a child or adult, and it relaxes randomly, quite frequently. As well as letting swallowed wind be released, these relaxations allow food (milk) to flow back into the oesophagus. For some babies – the 'happy chuckers' – this will just mean a few spills that don't seem to affect their wellbeing. At the other end of the spectrum, it can cause heartburn-like pain, abdominal pain and/or frequent vomiting, and can result in symptoms such as feeding issues and sudden waking and screaming. Of course, as babies are all individuals, symptoms will vary from one baby to another. For instance, constantly wanting to feed will soothe your baby's discomfort or he may need more feeds to make up for the milk he lost when he vomited. Another reason for constant feeding that may be attributed to reflux is that your baby is feeding to increase his sensory input. One way to meet baby's sensory needs is simply by carrying your baby in a carrier, going outside and engaging socially. This way, baby won't need to feed so voraciously to meet her natural needs.

Some babies may squirm and pull off the breast and may not feed well and while this may be a symptom of reflux discomfort, there can be other reasons so it can be helpful to check any feeding issues with a health professional such as a lactation consultant. Babies with reflux may also be diagnosed with low weight gain or breathing problems.

According to paediatric gastroenterologist Dr Bryan Vartabedian, author of *Colic Solved* and father of two babies with acid reflux, babies at extreme ends of this spectrum (happy chuckers or babies who are very unwell) are easily diagnosed, but the babies who are between extremes can be more challenging to treat, and even doctors can vary in their opinions as to when or how to treat baby heartburn.

Katrina had silent reflux (she didn't vomit) and colic. She was born at twenty-five weeks gestation. She came home ten days after full term, and for the first five weeks she was a really easy baby. Then, she became really unsettled and niggly after feeds. From seven to nine every night she would scream the house down. We worked as a team: my husband would make sure he was home from work and I would have dinner prepared early so we could be ready for her. We would walk, sing and massage for two hours, then she would just stop and go to sleep.

By six months, she was really niggly after feeds. The baby health nurse told us, 'It's just a baby thing,' and, 'Premmie babies can be a bit temperamental.' Her crying became so bad after each feed I felt I couldn't leave the house, but by the time I got to the doctor, she would be smiling. The doctor thought she may have been showing some early signs of cerebral palsy, so referred us to a paediatrician. He prescribed Mylanta, in a specific dose for her size, before each milk feed. I had tried Mylanta, but I hadn't given her enough, or at every feed. By following his instructions, within twenty-four to thirty-six hours her pain (and crying) was all over.

Angie

What can you do?

Firstly, have your baby checked by a doctor – your GP or paediatrician or ask for a referral to a paediatric gastroenterologist (if you are blown off, remember, you know your baby best; persist until you get answers to your baby's distress). A proper diagnosis can involve a treadmill of tests that often compound your baby's and your own distress. So, if other medical causes for your baby's distress have been ruled out, before you embark on invasive testing, consider whether his symptoms could be caused by conditions such as lactose overload (sometimes called foremilk intolerance), food intolerance, including reactions to foods that may pass through your breastmilk. Milk protein allergy can present with very similar symptoms to gastroesophageal reflux disease and is more likely if you have family history of allergies, asthma or eczema. If you are breastfeeding, these conditions can be simply addressed by eliminating offending foods from your own diet, rather than weaning: a child health nurse, dietician or lactation consultant can advise you. When considering changes to your own diet, also consider gut health as a factor in your baby's discomfort. Consult your health care provider about an appropriate probiotic for yourself and your baby. By taking a probiotic yourself, the benefits will be passed to your baby.

> I have a very fast letdown so my baby was often chok-
> ing and gagging at the start of his feeds. I also had a lot
> of foremilk which was causing him problems as his little
> tummy was forced to push through undigested milk
> which was then fermenting further down in his bowel
> and causing horrible gas pains. I got it under control by
> block feeding him for a few days (limiting baby to one
> side for period of three hours, i.e., if he needs to feed

*within that time, offer the same side). This settled my
oversupply. I now feed him off one breast only per feed,
and he is much easier to burp and isn't getting that
excruciating lower gut wind. I also noticed my son has
an upper-lip tie, while not severe enough to stop him
gaining huge amounts of weight, it affects his attachment so he can't get an airtight seal and sometimes
slips off or pinches my nipple because he can't flair his
top lip.*

Jess

Could it be tongue-tie?

Another thing to have checked is, could your baby have a physical issue such as a tongue- or lip tie. I have previously mentioned this but it's worth repeating in relation to how it can present with symptoms that may be confused with or diagnosed as reflux: a tongue-tie can affect your baby's ability to latch and suck effectively so he may suck in a lot of air as he feeds, causing discomfort both while he is feeding (Because it is hard work for him to stay attached to the breast) and afterwards as his tiny tummy is distended with wind. The baby with tongue- or lip tie may need to feed frequently due to a disordered ability to coordinate sucking, swallowing and breathing. This can contribute to a temporarily overabundant milk supply with symptoms of lactose overload and/or reflux. The good news is that if tongue-tie is the cause of your baby's reflux symptoms, this can be corrected quite simply either surgically or by laser, depending on the treating specialist, and will make feeding so much easier.

Positions to help

Until your baby's system matures, improving the positions he lies in during feeding and sleeping will be helpful to reduce his discomfort: holding your baby upright after feeds will aid digestion. However, young babies without much control of their abdominal or chest muscles tend to slump when placed in infant or car seats (reflux babies usually hate car seats). This increases pressure in their stomachs so worsens the reflux. Try using a baby carrier that supports your baby firmly in an upright position, comforts him and frees up your hands, or use an infant seat that reclines a bit.

Before you place your baby down to sleep, give him some upright time after feeds, so gravity can aid digestion – could you fall asleep on your back after drinking a milkshake? Hold your baby upright against you or wear him in a carrier that supports him upright for at least twenty minutes after a feed. One position that can be helpful for babies with reflux is placing your baby on his left side when you lie him down. This closes off the sphincter between the stomach and oesophagus and positions the sphincter above the stomach contents so that regurgitation is less likely. As a result, your baby may sleep more soundly on his left side – however as this is not advised by SIDS and Kids, please check with your health care provider and only do this when you are awake and able to watch that your baby doesn't roll onto his tummy while sleeping.

Meanwhile, please don't blame yourself for your high-needs baby. It's not your fault he cries (and cries!). You are never spoiling your baby by helping him feel safe and comfortable, and even if he cries despite your best efforts to help him, at least he will know you are there for him, through it all. This is an investment in his security and your relationship with your little one. And that will last long beyond these tough weeks and months.

12

Look after yourself

*'Without enough sleep, we all become
tall two-year-olds.'*

JoJo Jensen, *Dirt Farmer Wisdom*

When you have been attending to night-time waking, night after night, week after week, there is an enormous risk of parental burnout. The mother job spec doesn't include sick leave, or even much respite: it is a twenty-four-hour proposition. The most difficult part of being a parent is that small children are unpredictable, so no matter how well-organised you are, just when you have a pattern happening it changes as your child reaches a new developmental stage, gets a tooth or catches a bug. Even when things are going relatively smoothly (it's all relative isn't it?), there can be myriad interruptions so that your time is fragmented and you never seem to be able to finish a task in one attempt. It's not only about what you have to get done, another factor in how exhausted you can feel is hyper-vigilance: the constant state of awareness, focus and concentration that is so much a part of caring for babies and small children. Did you know that even the most easygoing baby will require nine hours of hands-on care a day? And the rest of the time you don't switch off from caring or planning and organising, so is it any wonder you feel as though you are riding an unstoppable treadmill? It is very easy to feel resentment towards your child, your partner or towards whoever you wish was giving you more help.

While it is easy to advise you to learn to go with the flow so that things don't seem so difficult, this is harder to put into practice. When you are exhausted, every little obstacle seems to be overwhelming, doesn't it? However, the best way to get through your days on very little sleep is to try to accept that this is how it is for now and to live one day at a time. This may sound like a big ask because it is probably totally contrary to the way you have coped before having a child. None of us likes to relinquish control and this is even more so when the world as we know it, or envisaged it would be, is spinning out of our grasp. But as you begin to surrender to the reality that babies do wake at night, you will be able to work out some practical survival strategies rather than simply wishing things were different and wasting energy on futile resentment or anger. You will also be present to experience your child as she is right now. After all, even though your job is challenging, you *can* enjoy being a mother – most days, at least.

Sleep is only an issue for us when I allow it to be. He is unable to go to sleep without being by my side (and sometimes on my breast), and if I get caught up in thoughts about the other things I should be doing instead (housework and other work), or would like to be doing (eating, showering, reading), I can get unhappy and annoyed about his dependence on me for sleep. The thought of just leaving the room and allowing him to cry has crossed my mind in those darker moments. But when I am able to switch off that internal chatter and just be with him, in the moment, while he falls asleep, it ceases to be an issue and I love watching him fall asleep.

Liz

Believe in yourself. Believe in your instincts. Write down at least one thing that you enjoy about your baby each day. And when she really gets up your nose pretend that she is somebody else's child – if only for a moment!

Abbey

Give me sleep

There probably is no better advice for any mother than the example given when we fly on planes – that you need to secure your own oxygen mask before you can help anybody else. If you are suffering from sleep deprivation, you need to take care of yourself so that you have some energy (and sanity) to care for your baby. Your first priority is to work out how you can make deposits into your sleep bank. While it may be unrealistic to expect one long sleep (even five hours in a row!), especially in the early weeks, it is important to take little rests whenever you can.

If possible, rest whenever your baby naps, rather than rushing around trying to get things done, especially in the first six weeks (and preferably three months) after birth when your body is in recovery mode. One way to manage this is to wear your baby in a carrier or wrap and get tasks done when he is awake. However, for many women napping during the day isn't a practical option, especially if you have other children. If you can, learn how to breastfeed lying down. Research shows that simply lying down to breastfeed increases prolactin, a breastfeeding hormone, and increases your milk supply, and this in itself may help your baby to sleep longer between feeds. Even if you have an older child who doesn't take naps, you can at least instil a quiet time each afternoon: as you either put your feet up and feed the baby or lie down and feed her, provide a quiet activity to engage your older child, or read stories to him.

> *Trying to synchronise a toddler and a baby to have a nap in the day at the same time is impossible! I find that sometimes in the early evening when I need to lie down with baby to feed him off to sleep (with hubby home from work) I often pass out into the deepest sleep for forty-five minutes. It really does recharge me for the rest of the evening.*
>
> **Sarah**

I often hear from mothers who complain that their baby takes his longer sleep during the early part of the evening – from about seven to midnight – then he wakes increasingly frequently as morning approaches. This is a fairly typical pattern for a young baby and some mothers would be grateful if their babies would at least take one longer sleep stretch whatever time this happens. The way to fill your sleep bank if this is your baby's pattern right now is to try to get to bed when your baby does at least two or three nights a week. This is a reasonable compromise so that you aren't missing out on couple time or 'me time' but you are taking care of your sleep needs. Hopefully you have a partner who can bathe and feed and put to bed your other children if the baby is not your only responsibility.

If you do take an afternoon siesta, guard this with your life. Making this a daily habit for at least the first three months will give you a great buffer against falling in a heap further down the track when you have a mobile baby to chase around. This may mean asserting to potential visitors that your health and wellbeing needs to be a priority. One diplomatic way around this is to hang out a sign with a notepad attached saying 'Mother and baby resting' so visitors can leave you a message if they do turn up while you are snoozing. They will soon get the hint to text or call before arriving.

If your partner has gone back to work soon after you have given birth, they can also get very tired combining work and a baby who wakes at night. Some partners take a shower with baby and a rest together when they get home from work so the other parent can get dinner started or have time out and be refreshed for the night shift (depending on baby's sleep patterns). You will need to work out your own way of sharing the load as a family. You may, for example, be able to take turns at sleeping in on weekends while one parent gets up to care for the baby. If your baby is an early riser, perhaps the partner who works outside the home could have a morning play or bath baby (or shower together, depending on baby's age) while mum sleeps. At risk of sounding incredibly old-fashioned, if your partner is the wage earner and you are the homemaker, do consider that he or she will also get very tired so it is generally unfair to expect them to be your sole support and completely take over home duties and baby care when they get home. Instead of risking resentment for either one of you, try to communicate how you can both enjoy the experience of being parents as you divide the workload – and sleep!

Perhaps the most important tip I could give you is to learn to pace yourself. When you have been feeling exhausted then you do have a good night it is tempting to use your newfound energy rushing around catching up. It is almost Mother Murphy's Law that this will backfire as you overdo things and crash again, or your baby has another bad night and you have nothing in reserve because you have used up your precious energy.

Pacing yourself also means prioritising invitations to events that may be tiring, and safeguarding your energy levels by having a nap in the afternoon before an evening outing, or possibly organising a babysitter for a few hours the next day so you can have a catch-up nap.

Baby is asleep, but you are awake

Even when your baby finally sleeps, you can find yourself wide awake with a mummy brain stream of consciousness of all the 'to dos' racing through your mind. Or, the crazy recurring voice in your head that does maths all night: 'If I get to sleep right now, I'll get two hours and forty-five minutes sleep before she next wakes.' You are so busy doing the mental arithmetic as the clock clicks over that eventually you are in a total panic because you *know* your baby will be awake in less than half an hour – so you just lie there frozen, frustrated and angry, waiting for the yell that says, she's awake. Relief: 'I can feed her and get back to sleep – I'll still get a couple of hours before the sun comes up. Better check the phone to make sure. Oh, I'll have a quick look at Facebook first . . .' And then, half an hour later, the room is getting lighter, the sounds of traffic are starting up, and before you know it, it's daybreak.

Sarah, a mother of a four-month-old, recently said, 'I am utterly exhausted and it is making me more anxious during the day. It's not my baby – she is sleeping pretty well, mostly only waking for one or two feeds – it's me. I find I no longer know how to switch off. And it's a vicious cycle. I am so overtired that my mind won't let me sleep. I sometimes go to sleep okay and get a block of two to three hours but once woken for the first feed, I am unable to go back to sleep.'

Sarah's experience seems to be fairly common to mums with young babies. However, not being able to sleep while your baby is sleeping peacefully can be a red flag that you may have a treatable medical illness such as postnatal depression, especially if your wakefulness is accompanied by other symptoms such as anxiety, teariness, mood swings and feelings of hopelessness. Of course some decent sleep may be all you need to make a difference to how you feel – it's a vicious cycle, isn't it? It is worth having a health check, especially your thyroids, and your vitamin D and iron levels.

> I found I couldn't sleep after both of my babies, even when they were sleeping. It turned out that my iron and vitamin-D levels were low. Taking a liquid iron twice a day made a huge difference.
>
> **Leah**

Once you have ruled out any underlying medical reasons for your mummy insomnia, here are some things to try to get those essential zzz's:

- Prepare your sleep environment: switch off screens an hour before bed – and banish them from the bedroom. The light from devices and computer screens affects the brain's production of melatonin, your natural sleep-inducing hormone. Dim lighting as you read or relax before bed will help trigger melatonin production.

- Banish clocks from the bedroom: or place them where you can't see the time, to avoid midnight mathematics (or, how long have I been awake?)

- Create a gentle bedtime routine for yourself: have a nice warm bath or shower – one trigger for sleep is a slight drop in core body temperature so after a warm bath, as your body cools, you will naturally begin to feel drowsy and more relaxed (works for kids too).

- Make a warm drink and take it to bed to sip. A snack of carbs will help release tryptophan (bananas are rich in tryptophan), a precursor to serotonin, a relaxing hormone.
- Practise deep breathing and/or a guided relaxation to help you switch off and enter more relaxed sleep.
- Download a talking book or some podcasts to listen to. If you find yourself awake after you have fed your baby, instead of focusing on sleep, pop in earplugs and listen to your download. This will distract your busy mind and override your anxiety. Rather than keeping yourself awake, you will actually find you miss the plot because you dozed off. This is much better than missing sleep!

Foods to boost your energy

When we are tired we often neglect our diets, but nutrition is one area where you really do need to get your priorities sorted. Having breakfast should be your first priority every day: you can give yourself a head start in the energy stakes and maintain energy levels well into the afternoon by eating a nutritious breakfast that includes some protein. Rolled oats (yes, that's good old-fashioned porridge!) have been cited as a food to help fight depression, perhaps because they maintain blood sugar levels, and drops in blood sugar levels are associated with mood swings.

When you are tired and never seem to have a free hand or spare moment, it is very easy to reach for snacks that provide a sugar hit, especially when you hit the proverbial wall late in the afternoon – I call this 'three-thirty-itis' – but this creates a vicious cycle: once the sugar fix wears off and your blood sugar levels drop, you hit rock bottom much more quickly than if you had taken a few extra minutes to eat something healthy. Also, consider that quick hits of chocolate or caffeine in the afternoon may be keeping your baby awake in the evening as he fills up on the chemicals and caffeine through your breastmilk.

Next time you are shopping, add some healthy protein or complex carbohydrate snacks to your basket: canned salmon or sardines (these are high in DHA, an omega-3 fatty acid that will nourish your nervous system), cheese, avocado, eggs (hard boil and keep in the fridge for when hunger strikes), wholegrain bread and cereals, yoghurt, green leafy salad vegetables (these have a natural calming effect due to their high magnesium content), fresh or dried fruit and nuts.

Drink plenty of water. Fatigue is one of the first and most common signs of dehydration. Drink whenever you feed your baby and at mealtimes, and carry a water bottle when you go out. Speaking of which, getting outside each day, even for a walk around the block, will not only help your baby sleep better, but it will boost your own endorphins and help you build up stamina.

It's only appearances

Isn't it easy to feel intimidated by the endless home and beauty makeover shows on television? It may help to remind yourself that it takes a whole heap of stylists and labour – not to mention energy – to keep up those sorts of appearances. Sadly, when we are tired and at our most vulnerable, we are likely to feel stressed by clutter and mess all around us. If you can afford some hired help, see it as an investment in your family's wellbeing. Even having your house thoroughly cleaned just once, or seeing the bottom of the ironing basket occasionally can give you a boost. If you can't afford regular help, try one-off sanity savers such as dropping a few shirts into the drycleaners to be ironed or buying a ready-cooked meal from your local deli.

There are a few other shortcuts that might help:

- **Work around the rhythms of your baby.** Prepare dinner early in the day, so you aren't stressed when arsenic hour arrives and you have a grizzly baby or grumpy toddler to contend with. Let a slow cooker become your new best friend; a rice cooker will do risotto that you don't need to watch. Prepare in bursts: chop vegies in the morning or through the day and throw it all in later to cook. Bonus: you can snack on the chopped veggies as you go, or use some of the dinner onions and peppers to make yourself a simple scrambled egg for lunch. Make double batches of food and freeze for difficult days.
- **Simplify mealtimes.** Work out a few simple meals and stock your cupboards with the ingredients so

that you'll be able to whip up a meal quickly on busy days. (Or cook extra and freeze leftovers as standby meals.) Serve fresh fruit instead of desserts. Eat some meals on paper plates. Choose one night as takeaway night or have a baked-bean dinner occasionally – add a glass of milk, some wholegrain bread and fruit and you have four food groups!

- **Plan simple toddler play.** Before you go to bed, set up an activity for your toddler so he engages in his surprise and gives you a bit of time to get your morning started. You may like to google 'busy bags' for some creative ideas beyond playdough, blocks or stickers, although these are all engaging activities, especially if you add some props such as dough cutters and pasta noodles to poke into Play Dough, or little plastic animals or people and cars to drive around the block buildings. And if it's a fine day, a great activity that engages toddlers is to give them a shallow bucket or bowl of water and a house-sized paintbrush and let them paint the fence or steps while you sit and watch as you feed your baby.

- **Make fewer shopping trips.** Keep a notepad in the kitchen and jot down what you need as it occurs to you or make lists on your phone then just make a weekly or fortnightly shopping trip rather than racing out every day. This will save you money as well as time. To save time and energy trudging the supermarket aisles (unless you find this therapeutic), why not order your groceries online through one of the large supermarket chains, or email your shopping list to your partner or someone who is coming to visit and let them bring the groceries home.

- **Divide your workload.** Don't knock yourself out trying to clean the whole house from top to bottom while baby is asleep, only to find you are exhausted by the time he wakes up. Plan one large job each day, such as cleaning the fridge or the bathroom, or tidying one cupboard or bookshelf. By the end of the week it will all get done and if it doesn't, as long as choking hazards are picked up, no small children will suffer because they lived in an untidy house; they won't remember whether they wore clothes that were ironed or not and they won't give a toss if they ate cheese on toast and fruit for dinner some nights or if they ate a picnic dinner in the bath – this saves clean-ups as the mess goes down the plughole, you are multi-tasking so it saves time plus everyone has fun!
- **Pay bills over the internet.** This gives you more flexibility for managing time. Set up auto-payments of bills via direct debit with utilities such as gas, electricity and phone companies. And keeping stamps, envelopes and parcel bags at home is always handy to avoid post office queues.
- **Tidy up once, late in the day.** If you have a toddler it can be frustrating to try to keep things orderly all day. One late-afternoon tidy will help make you feel relaxed and less flustered as you face the evening rush. It may also prevent friction with partners who

have an aversion to coming home to apparent (or total) chaos. Aim for efficiency: walk around with a supermarket carry bag or a basket and collect everything that is scattered. Deliver the contents in one trip, rather than repeatedly running the length of the house to put each object away separately. Older kids can collect their own junk from the bag. Get all children (of any age, who can walk and talk) to help with tidy-ups. Make it a game at first: they will never know the difference, as long as you smile! Kids under six learn best by imitation, so work with them rather than expecting them to follow orders.

- **Wear baby in a carrier as you do chores.** He'll enjoy the ride and the view, and you'll get extra jobs done. And then you'll feel freer to rest when he sleeps.

- **Provide a haven from the chaos.** Keeping small corners attractive, or one room tidy, can provide sanctuary when most of the house is in a muddle. Little things like fresh flowers look cheerful. Burning essential oils (keep the burner away from small children) makes for a calm and nurturing environment.

- **Delegate.** Your partner and family members aren't mind-readers. Ask for help when you need it (and remember to say thanks, even if you feel it was the other person's duty anyway).

What about me?

I have realised lately that I have lost myself. All I am now is a mum and a worker (in my job) and the me that was once there is long gone. I spend all of my time focused on my family and I don't take time for myself, participate in hobbies or even really see many of my friends anymore.

Jane

Being everything to your baby and watching her grow into a unique little person is exciting and wondrous and while there are moments of absolute joy, the intensity of meeting everyone else's needs can ever so sneakily over-take your own needs for self-care. Then, almost suddenly it seems, feelings of being overwhelmed and lost can hit.

I was zoning out on the couch thinking, I can't do this. I'm a half-assed mother, friend, wife. Am I horrible to want a hot cup of coffee once a week? Eat a sandwich without children crawling on me? Pee when I need to? The TV was on the documentary channel, it was about a lioness and her cub who hadn't eaten in two days and it was getting critical for both. She made a kill, the mother, and ate it. She didn't give any to the cub. At first I was revolted. Then the narrator said, 'She must or else she won't be able to hunt for bigger game to share with her cub and they will surely both perish.' And, sure enough, she then made a big-ger kill for the both of them. It was like a sign for me.

Sonia

It's easy to be swallowed up by motherhood. Babies and small children need to be taken care of – that's what we sign up for; some little ones need more care than others and we don't always have the support that would make things easier. We know that if we don't stay on top of things and pre-empt the tougher times (think, arsenic hour when you don't have dinner planned), it can all go to hell in a handbasket in no time. And crawling back out of that hellish handbasket can take more energy than if we didn't let things go there in the first place. So, we become the cog that keeps the wheels turning. Until one day we realise we are on autopilot, putting one foot in front of the other hoping that when we look up there isn't a wall in front of us. Or, like Jane, we realise we have lost our own sense of self.

Ideally, we would all look up before we hit the proverbial wall, we would realise it isn't selfish to take care of ourselves, that you can be a good mother without completely sacrificing your own needs for even basic self-care – I would be a millionaire if I had just one dollar for the number of women who have told me, 'I don't even have time for a shower every day.' But the all-consuming nature of caring for babies and children and running a home means that self-neglect happens so slowly, over time, that we shrink into a smaller and smaller space until there is no 'me' left. Like the lioness, if you don't nourish yourself, you won't be able to sustain your own energy or health.

Although nurturing yourself will probably mean very simple things at first – and if you have a newborn, it will probably include your baby – it is absolutely essential that you exercise, that you nourish your body with fresh, healthy foods, and that you surround yourself with positive support. It's also important to speak up about your needs, especially with your partner to work out how you can carve out some 'me time' otherwise it looks as though you are doing just fine.

- **Schedule one activity a week.** What did you enjoy before you had a baby? Sport? Craft? Cooking? Try a class at a community house that offers babysitting or join a gym with childcare. Or, join your partner up at a gym and get them to take the kids to the crèche there so you can have some quiet time at home alone – and don't spend that time cleaning!
- **Meet up with a friend who also has kids.** Laugh together, vent together and take turns watching the little ones so you each get to sip a hot cuppa. Or do something useful like cooking some meals together. Then you can have more 'me time' because you will go home with meals ready for the next few days.
- **Start a gratitude list** – and share with friends (text your lists to each other). Before you go to bed each night, list the things you are grateful for today. This will help you release negative thoughts and interrupt the cycle of despair as it sets you up for a positive mindset to start to the next day.
- **Ditch the stereotypes of a 'good mother'.** Your little ones are the most accurate barometers of your own stress and discontent. They deserve a happy, healthy mum and you can achieve this without neglecting their needs, or your own.

*As a 'mother' of six (two dogs, a fifteen-month-old son,
a four-year-old daughter, a fifteen-year-old stepson
and my husband, in no particular order), who also
works full-time and is a self-confessed control-freak, I
have found that even five minutes a day to myself helps
keep the calm. This might be spent catching up on my
junk mail when everyone has gone to bed, or having a
long, hot shower and some thinking time before the
'kids' get up . . .*

*I also schedule appointments with myself, for time
to be me, not mum, for a while. Coffee with the girls,
a massage, a haircut all deserve my attention as much
as my family does, as without them I feel out of touch,
tired and not able to cope with the workload at hand.*

*When I look after me, well, I look after my 'kids'
well, too. Nurturing starts from the inside.*

Mandie

*Being rather busy with two children (my youngest a
very clingy fourteen-month-old), finding an opportunity to self-nurture is a rarity, although being able to
combine mothering and nurturing myself is more realistic for me. I love being a mother, and find that time
away from my baby feels unnatural (especially when
he is a boobaholic!), so being able to go for long walks
with my baby in a sling or in a pram is relaxing and
enjoyable for us both. At home, when my husband and
older son are home from work and school, I am able to
utilise their hands and energy for entertaining baby, so
I can have a soak in the bath. And late at night I love*

sitting up in bed, baby and husband asleep nestled up close to me, and quietly reading a book, with a hand resting on my baby. Maybe as my youngest gets older I will enjoy going out for coffee with a girlfriend, but for now combining mothering and self-nurturing feels right for me!

Nicole

Networking the mother 'hood'

Joining the mother 'hood' offers a new dimension to the concept of networking. Although it probably won't help you raise any glass ceilings, your network of mothers may prevent you from sliding into a downward spiral towards isolation and despair. A support group can be an invaluable source of help and information, especially if you find your parenting style at odds with others around you or if you are feeling pressure to deal with your wakeful baby in ways that don't feel right to you. You could hit the jackpot with your new mothers' group or you may need to search around to meet women who are more supportive of your mothering style.

It is also a great idea to create your own network of people who can be of specific help. It can come as an enormous shock just how vulnerable you can feel on very little sleep and how hard it can be to ask for help, or even to consider who might be helpful when you are at the end of your tether, so it is best to work out who you would like in your network long before you are sleep deprived and in despair. Do this together with your partner but be warned that it can make for a few surprises about each other's perceptions of your friends and theirs.

To start, list five people you and your partner feel you could call on for help. Next, write down the kinds of support you would find most helpful, then set out to find it. Your list should include a neighbour you can call in an emergency, an experienced mother who will offer support without judging you and several back-up people. To this list, add emergency contacts such as your family doctor, a local hospital, and the maternal and child health helpline. You might also want access to breastfeeding help, emotional support, a supermarket or fruit shop that delivers, a local takeaway restaurant, a cleaner, a dogwasher, an ironing lady, a lawnmowing company – whatever will help you. Keep your list of helpers (with contact details) on a wall where you can easily see it in an emergency.

Many parents find support on the internet. It isn't the same as a face-to-face chat or a real shoulder to cry on and the advice you will receive can be questionable at times, but it can be comforting to know that there is a whole community of sleepless parents who can offer commiseration even at three in the morning, and it can be amazing to discover that parents all over the world have similar concerns and feelings. If this appeals to you, find some websites or social media communities that support your parenting style and provide good health information. Consider subscribing to relevant online newsletters that will boost your mindset and make you feel good about your parenting role. Conversely, unsubscribe to newsletters that undermine your parenting style or your confidence.

Although it can be helpful to vent your feelings of frustration to faceless people on the internet or a telephone helpline, one of the most difficult things for most of us is to ask for practical help from friends and family. Ironically, a new baby is like a magnet and most people feel privileged to be invited to share this special time. Can you call your mum, sister or aunt to come and stay for a few days or can you go and stay with a family member who will support you as you catch up on some much-needed rest? Please don't worry about feeling judged because you aren't coping. If they have had babies themselves, they will understand. You may even be giving them an opportunity to speak about how hard it was for them in their own early days.

If you give your loved ones specific tasks, they will usually feel more comfortable about offering help than if they feel that they may be intruding. Perhaps create a help-list roster before you have your baby: if you feel you couldn't do this yourself, you could supply a list of suspects to a good friend and let her organise the roster for you. One couple I interviewed asked their baby shower guests for help instead of gifts. They asked each guest to bring two notes – one with a piece of advice and one with a pledge of help.

Mind your health

Having a baby places an enormous stress on your body and mind, but even though we acknowledge this, the extreme exhaustion of new parenthood is a huge shock. According to Australian GP Dr Oscar Serrallach, lethargy, memory disturbances (mummy brain), and poor energy levels, among other symptoms, are not just because being a parent is hard but can be due to a condition he calls 'postnatal depletion'. In an interview I conducted with Dr Serrallach, he emphasised that the physical process of growing a baby exacts a significant toll on a mother's body as it taps into your levels of essential nutrients such as iron, zinc, vitamin B12, vitamin B9, iodine and selenium stores, along with omega-3 fats like DHA and specific amino acids

If you are overwhelmed by tiredness, especially to the point of crying, and this feeling isn't relieved by extra rest or has gone on for more than two weeks, do see your doctor for a check-up. You may be trying to push through tiredness when there is a medical condition that could be treated.

Ask to have your thyroid, iron and vitamin-D levels checked: low iron levels or thyroid disorders are both reasonably common in the postnatal period and many of us have low vitamin D levels regardless of pregnancy or child-bearing status. These can all cause extreme tiredness and low vitamin D can affect our immunity and make us more prone to illness – and mothers don't get sick leave! Thyroid disorders can also cause other symptoms such as sensitivity to cold, anxiety and dry skin.

Also, if you are having mood swings or feel so inadequate that your baby deserves another mother, or that your family would be better off without you, you may be suffering from postnatal depression. This is nothing to feel afraid or embarrassed about – postnatal depression is an illness, not a reflection of your coping skills, and it is treatable. Are you wondering, where is the line between the normal maze of maternal emotions and the black tunnel of depression? The difficult thing is that most women don't simply wake up one morning with postnatal depression. Although the illness can present during pregnancy, immediately after birth or in the next few weeks, it can also develop slowly over several months. Symptoms may include mood swings, sleep disturbances that are unrelated to your baby's waking, chronic exhaustion or hyperactivity, uncontrollable crying, extreme irritability, loss of memory or concentration, anxiety or panic.

The debilitating exhaustion that is a characteristic of depressive illness will affect your ability to enjoy your baby and may also affect your ability to respond appropriately which could result in a vicious cycle of an unsettled, wakeful baby and increasing stress for you. This is a quality-of-life issue so please discuss your thoughts and feelings honestly with your doctor or maternal and child health nurse if you are experiencing extreme exhaustion or irritability. If you feel that your concerns are not being taken seriously, take a good friend or your partner to the doctor with you. (Also, be reassured, there are medications that can safely be taken for postnatal depression while you are breastfeeding.)

Call an expert

It may help to call in a detached expert who can offer some settling tips, reassurance or even some nurturing for you so that you regain your energy and get your life back on track. You can get help from the range of support groups in the resources section at the back of this book or you can seek other professional help. You may find the following people helpful.

Maternal and child health nurses

You don't have to attend your local clinic if you prefer a nurse in another area – some will have extra qualifications. Baby health nurses are well informed about infant development. A good nurse will be able to help with feeding and sleep issues as well as being able to support you with your own health and adjustment to motherhood. Many organise groups for new mothers where you will meet others with babies the same age as yours and this can be very reassuring as you discover that your baby's sleep behaviour (and your own tiredness) is quite normal. Your nurse is part of a large network of other resources so she can refer you elsewhere if you have concerns about any aspect of your baby's development, including sleep, which she cannot address. It will also help to keep an after-hours number handy. Even though the after-hours nurse won't be the person who is familiar with your baby she will have lots of experience and expertise about babies, and it is reassuring to know you can contact a professional in the middle of the night.

Midwives

Whether you had a midwife in private practice for your baby's birth or whether you had your baby in hospital, you can call and ask for help either from your birth midwife or the hospital where your baby was born. The hospital is staffed around the clock, and even if the person you speak to doesn't know you, they will be able to offer some tips if you are in the middle of a crisis.

Lactation consultants

Lactation consultants are allied health professionals who offer support and specialist breastfeeding assistance. They are often employed by hospitals, either in maternity wards, mother–baby units or in breastfeeding clinics where mothers and babies can spend a few hours or a whole day for help with breastfeeding problems. (Many maternal and child health nurses and independent midwives are also certified lactation consultants.) Some lactation consultants work in private practice and will visit families at home to help with feeding and settling issues – this is a boon if you are having difficulty finding the letterbox, or if you know you would be a danger on the roads in your sleep-deprived state.

To make sure that the person you consult is offering proficient advice, check that she is a qualified International Board Certified Lactation Consultant and a member of a recognised professional body – members of Lactation Consultants of Australia and New Zealand or of the International Lactation Consultants Association are internationally certified professionals bound by a code of ethics and standard of practice.

Mother–baby units

Mother–baby units may be part of the public health system (which means you won't have to pay for a stay) or attached to private maternity units (which may be covered by health insurance), and while some offer day stays to observe you feed and settle your baby and offer a few pointers, others book you in with your baby for several days which can be an opportunity to relax and feel nurtured as you work at solving your baby's sleep puzzle.

Some mother–baby units take a very gentle approach and encourage you to respond to your baby at all times, others will implement a fairly rigid 'one size fits all' controlled crying regime. They may use a less confronting name for whatever they do but it can still be a version of leaving your baby to cry. You will probably be at a stage of peak vulnerability before you check into a mother–baby unit (many have considerable waiting lists and some health insurance companies are not overly supportive about this option) so you may find it difficult to resist harsh methods once you are actually in an unfamiliar environment. It may help to assess exactly what your objectives are (and those of the unit) before you discover you have booked into a 'baby boot camp'. Always remember, this is your baby, you don't have to do anything that doesn't feel right for you. You can negotiate with staff and expect to have explanations for anything they advise. And, if it's not for you, you are free to leave.

Doulas

The role of a doula is to help *you*, not to solve your baby's feeding or sleeping problems. The word doula is derived from a Greek word meaning mother's servant. This pretty much explains the role of a doula who may offer services ranging from birth support to practical postnatal help. A postnatal doula can be the next best thing to having your mum to help. And, because you are paying her, you can say what you need done without feeling you are imposing. A doula can come in for a few hours to 'pack you together' and watch your baby while you catch up on some uninterrupted sleep. She can cook a meal, hang out washing and make you a cuppa – just like your own mum.

Although there are no national standards for doula training, there are several training providers so you will need to do your homework and ask what is offered and what qualifications your prospective doula has. Some doulas will have extra qualifications or experience and will offer services accordingly, such as breastfeeding counselling or massage.

Baby sleep consultants

There are baby sleep consultants who will come to your home. This is where you need to really take care. There is a plethora of online courses in baby sleep training that give their graduates certificates; there are baby sleep trainers with no qualifications in early childhood or infant health; there are baby sleep trainers who will come to your home overnight to teach your baby to sleep but who have been found sleeping on the sofa while the baby has been left to cry.

Consider, this person is coming into your home, she is meeting your child, she is advising you on your baby's wellbeing. You need to be very clear about what you need and what you are prepared to allow before you hire this person. Ask, what qualifications do you have? Check what these actually mean and what the scope of the training is. For instance, if you have a breastfed baby, can this person assess your baby's feeding to see whether this is impacting your baby's sleep? Will this person do a history that includes any health issues for you and your baby or does she see sleep as a behavioral problem? If she suspects an issue that requires help from another professional, such as infant reflux, possible allergies, feeding problems or developmental issues, will she refer you to an appropriate resource? Will she support and respect you and your beliefs? If she gives you explanations that sound reasonable but have you doubting yourself, try the filter: is it safe? Is it respectful? Does it feel right? And if anything feels stressful for you or your baby, ditch it. Remember, you are the expert on your child.

What you do matters

In our roles as men and women, we are encouraged to give ourselves over completely to our careers, to our relationships or to 'finding ourselves'. We are encouraged to slot our parental role around all of these other – read, more important – things in our lives. Our culture places very little value on nurturing, or the fulfilment that we can experience as we cherish our little ones: at every turn we are bombarded with messages that imply we can 'have it all' – from a good night's sleep to an unaltered waist-line – if we simply follow one method or another; that we can have convenient babies and children who will not change our lives and that this is an admirable goal.

It is this very pressure and denial of the value of our nurturing role that makes it all so challenging. Right now, it may seem overwhelming that you could possibly continue giving of your body, your mind and your soul. As you stagger through a fog of sleeplessness, it is likely that you will experience ugly feelings of resentment and anger, or worse. This is perfectly normal in a world that neither honours nor supports parenting as valued work.

However, as you struggle to balance your own needs with the intensive demands of your infant, it is important to maintain perspective and to understand the significance of your nurturing role to your child and your own identity. Having a child is a privilege. A baby is a gift of life and it is up to each of us lucky enough to share this tiny life to make it worthwhile – to nurture and grow this little being, teaching it how to love and to love life. As you teach your baby that he is loved and worthwhile and special, he will also teach you about pure, unconditional love. For that is what you will find in your heart when you surrender to your feelings and allow yourself to connect unreservedly with the tiny person in your arms – day and night.

As you mutter the mantra for when the going gets

tough, 'this too shall pass', I promise it will. For now, it might help to think of your lifetime as a length of cord. Imagine tying a knot in your cord for each decade and you will see that, as lifetimes go, the time that your tiny child needs you at night is really not that long. I hope that instead of wishing away the hours that you are awake at night, you can cherish each precious moment with your little one. All too soon, your baby will have grown out of your arms and out of your bed, and these nights of holding her close will be just a distant memory.

Useful contacts and resources

ALLERGIES AND FOOD INTOLERANCE

Food Intolerance Network

fedup.com.au

Sue Dengate, author of books on allergies and food intolerance, including *Fed Up* and *The Failsafe Cookbook*, offers a wealth of information and resources including articles, parent stories, links, a list of food additives and a free newsletter.

BREASTFEEDING

Australian Breastfeeding Association

breastfeeding.asn.au

The Australian Breastfeeding Association offers a range of services including classes for mothers-to-be who intend to breastfeed their baby, and support for mothers and babies.

24-hour breastfeeding helpline
1800 686 268

Lactation Consultants Australia and New Zealand (LCANZ)

lcanz.org
Health professionals offering breastfeeding advice and information. Many hospitals have midwives who are certified lactation consultants. There are also private lactation consultants who offer home visits.

GASTRIC REFLUX

Distressed Infants Support Association (DISA) of Vic Inc

(03) 9786 8568

Vomiting Infants Support Association (VISA) of New South Wales

(02) 4324 7062

MASSAGE

Pinky McKay's Baby Massage DVD

pinkysbabymassage.com

A beautiful guide to massaging your baby.

Infant Massage Australia

infantmassage.org.au

Directory of instructors and links to international sites.

MULTIPLE BIRTH

Australian Multiple Birth Association Inc. (AMBA)

amba.org.au

A volunteer organisation providing support and resources to families and/or carers of twins, triplets and more.

MUSIC FOR RELAXATION AND MEDITATION

Music for Dreaming

musicfordreaming.com

Classical music played by members of the Melbourne Symphony Orchestra in one continuous piece in 3/4 rhythm – the natural rhythm of the human heartbeat; it's used in many hospital nurseries and intensive care units.

PARENTING INFORMATION AND SUPPORT

Beyond Blue

beyondblue.org.au/the-facts/postnatal-depression

PANDA (Perinatal Anxiety & Depression Australia)

panda.org.au
1300 726 306

How Is Dad Going?

howisdadgoing.org
National helpline for men affected by perinatal depression and anxiety, whether you have a partner with PND or whether you are suffering anxiety or depression yourself. Helpline is also via PaNDA, 1300 726 306.

Raising Children Network

raisingchildren.net.au
Parenting resource for all stages from pregnancy to newborns to teens, including lists of national parenting helplines.

SIDS and Kids

sidsandkids.org/safe-sleeping
Safe sleeping information, including safe-sleep guidelines and product safety.

GENERAL HELPLINES

Alcohol and Drug Information Services (ADIS)

1800 422 599
(02) 9361 8000 (Sydney metro)
24 hours, 7 days

Child Care Access Hotline

1800 670 305
133 677 (TTY service for people with a hearing/
speech impairment), 8 a.m. to 6 p.m., Monday
to Friday

Child Wise National Child Abuse Prevention Helpline

1800 991 099
9 a.m. to 5 p.m., Monday to Friday

Family Relationship Advice Line

1800 050 321
8 a.m. to 8 p.m., Monday to Friday and
10 a.m. to 4 p.m. on Saturdays

Lifeline

131 114

NEW ZEALAND RESOURCES

La Leche League New Zealand
lalecheleague.org/LLLNZ
Breastfeeding information and support.

Parents Centre
parentscentre.org.nz
Pregnancy, childbirth, postnatal and parenting education programs and support offered through a strong support network of fifty centres around the country. Magazine *Kiwi Parent*.

Plunket New Zealand
plunket.org.nz
0800 933 922
Professional child and family support services for the development, health and wellbeing of children under five.

Further reading

BOOKS

Douglas, P., *The Discontented Little Baby Book*, UQP, St Lucia, 2014.

Garth, M., *Moonbeam: A Book of Meditations for Children*, HarperCollins, Melbourne 1997.

Gerhardt, S., *Why Love Matters: How Affection Shapes a Baby's Brain*, Routledge, London, 2004.

La Leche League International, *The Womanly Art of Breastfeeding*, Ballantine Books, New York, 2010.

La Leche League International, *Sweet Sleep: Nighttime and Naptime Strategies for the Breastfeeding Family*, Pinter & Martin, London, 2014.

McKay, P., *Parenting By Heart*, Penguin Books (Australia), Melbourne, 2011.

McKay, P., *100 Ways to Calm the Crying*, Penguin Books (Australia), Melbourne, 2008.

McKay, P., *Toddler Tactics*, Penguin Books (Australia), Melbourne, 2008.

Minchin, M., *Milk Matters, Infant Feeding and Immune Disorder*, Milk Matters Pty Ltd, Melbourne, Australia, 2015.

Odent, M., *Primal Health*, Clairview Books, London, 2002.

Sunderland, M., *The Science of Parenting*, DK, London, 2006.

Van der Rijt, H. & Plooij, F., *The Wonder Weeks*, Kiddy World Promotions, BV, 2003.

There is also a 'Wonder Weeks' app that supports this book on child development so you can track your baby's 'leaps'.

WEBSITES

Pinky McKay

pinkymckay.com
Yes, this is my site! Loads of evidence-based information and practical support including my blog, free newsletter, books, live seminars, teleseminars and my Baby Massage DVD. For breastfeeding information, see my blog at beautifulbreastfeeding.com

Association for Prenatal and Perinatal Psychology and Health (APPAH)

birthpsychology.com

Australian Association of Infant Mental Health Inc. (AAIMHI)

aaimhi.org

AAIMHI is a national organisation of professionals from many fields who work with infants and their families towards improving professional and community recognition that infancy is a critical time for psycho-social development. See their policy statements on controlled crying and responding to infants.

Mother–Baby Behavioral Sleep Laboratory

cosleeping.nd.edu

Professor McKenna, the director of the Mother–Baby Behavioral Sleep Lab at the University of Notre Dame, Indiana, is an acclaimed expert in the areas of infant sleep, breastfeeding and Sudden Infant Death Syndrome.

Infant Sleep Information Source (ISIS)

isisonline.org.uk

Evidence-based information on infant sleep for parents and health professionals. The ISIS website draws on the combined experience of Professor Helen Ball and her team at the Durham University Parent–Infant Sleep Lab, and senior representatives from La Leche League, NCT, and UNICEF UK Baby Friendly Initiative, all being organisations working directly in the fields of parent-support and health professional training in the UK.

La Leche League International

llli.org

The leading international breastfeeding organisation. Information, support and groups supporting mothering through breastfeeding in over fifty countries.

Evolutionary Parenting

evolutionaryparenting.com

Tracy Cassels, PhD in developmental psychology, is the founder and primary writer on this site. Evidence-based information on the science and importance of attachment and evolutionary parenting. Informative articles on infant sleep, breastfeeding and emotional development.

Kangaroo Care

kangaroomothercare.com

A method of care for all newborns, but in particular for premature babies, with three components: skin-to-skin contact; exclusive breastfeeding; support to the mother–infant dyad.

Dr Sarah Buckley

sarahbuckley.com

Author of *Gentle Birth, Gentle Mothering*, GP Sarah Buckley provides inspiring and meticulously researched articles on birth and parenting, including sleep.

Ask Dr Sears

askdrsears.com

Attachment parenting guru William Sears and his sons (all of whom are paediatricians) offer evidence-based information about all aspects of parenting, including co-sleeping.

Attachment Parenting International

attachmentparenting.org

Educational materials, research information, consultative, referral and speaker services to promote parenting practices that create strong, healthy emotional bonds between children and their parents. These practices nurture a child's need for trust, empathy and affection, providing a lifelong foundation for healthy, enduring relationships.

Gentle Parenting

gentleparenting.co.uk

Information with a focus on empathic, compassionate parenting for all parents, no matter how they feed their baby, whether they use a buggy or a sling, whether they use a cot or bedshare, whether they birth at home or in hospital and whether they are pregnant with their first child or have a brood of six children.

Acknowledgements

I would like to give a big thank you to all the parents who have shared their experiences in *Sleeping like a Baby*. I am sure your stories will help validate others who are struggling with the immense pressure to have a 'good' baby (read: a baby who self-settles and sleeps 'all night').

Sleeping Like a Baby includes a wide range of evidence-based information. I owe a huge debt of gratitude to the researchers in infant sleep who acknowledge and affirm the relationship between sleep, infant feeding, mother/baby attachment and infant brain development. I am especially grateful for the works of Helen Ball, Nils Bergman and James McKenna; Kathleen Kendall-Tackett, Tracy Cassels, Michel Odent, Robin Grille, Darcia Narvaez, Diana West, and Maureen Minchin for their meticulous and passionate work.

A big thank you, too, to my brilliant agent Jacinta di Mase for her unending commitment and support. Also to the team at Penguin Australia for their care and concern, especially Clementine Edwards for being such an easy editor to work with.

My work is a reflection of the support and love I received from my own mentors as I found my way through the haze of sleepless nights when I was a young mother: my mother, who said I slept with her when I was a newborn; my first GP, who set me straight when, as a sleep-deprived new mother, I begged him for 'something to make my baby sleep'; and the wonderful women of La Leche League in Cambridge and Hamilton, New Zealand, especially Yvonne Foreman. Through their modelling and practical support, these wise women taught me so much about responding to babies – day and night!

Last, but certainly not least, thank you to my own babies (some of whom slept more than others!) for teaching me my greatest lessons about patience, flexibility and unconditional love, and to my husband for supporting our night-time parenting.

Index